50 Bread Baking Recipes 2021

Secret Recipes of the Masters of Bread!

Table of Contents

INTRODUCTION 4
BASIC BABKA 6
SWEET CHALLAH BREAD 9
IRRESISTIBLE WHOLE WHEAT CHALLAH 12
MOST AMAZING CHALLAH 14
MIRIAM'S NOT-SO-SECRET CHALLAH 16
SY'S CHALLAH 18
SHABBAT CHALLAH 20
MICHELL JENNY'S CHALLAH 22
EKMEK TURKISH BREAD 24
SYRIAN BREAD 26
SERENDIPITY BREAD 28
BAZLAMA - TURKISH FLAT BREAD 30
PEPPY'S PITA BREAD 32
FOCACCIA ALLA GENOVESE 34
NONI AFGHANI 36
LEPINJA (SERBIAN FLATBREAD) 38
NAAN 40
CHEF JOHN'S PITA BREAD 42
LONG-FERMENTATION BREAD 44
NO-KNEAD WHOLE WHEAT BREAD WITH SORGHUM FLOUR 46
ARTISAN NO-KNEAD BREAD WITH AMARANTH 48
DUTCH OVEN CARAWAY RYE BREAD 50
RUSTIC BREAD 52
ENGLISH MUFFIN LOAVES 54
GLUTEN-FREE SOURDOUGH RAISIN BREAD 56
NO-KNEAD SKILLET OLIVE BREAD 58
SLOW COOKER BREAD 60
NO-KNEAD COUNTRY BREAD 62
BETTER-THAN-BAKERY NO-KNEAD SOURDOUGH 64
CHEF JOHN'S WHOLE WHEAT CIABATTA 66

PIZZA BREAD	68
GLUTEN-FREE CHEESE AND HERB PIZZA CRUST	70
WHOLE WHEAT AND HONEY PIZZA DOUGH	72
AMAZING WHOLE WHEAT PIZZA CRUST	74
VALENTINO'S PIZZA CRUST	76
GRILL DOUGH	78
NO-YEAST PIZZA CRUST	80
COLLEEN'S POTATO CRESCENT ROLLS	82
POTATO BREAD RECIPE 2	84
CRUSTY POTATO BREAD	86
POTATO ROSEMARY BREAD	88
CLARE'S WHOLE WHEAT POTATO BREAD	90
ZADI'S POTATO BREAD	92
HIGH RISE DINNER ROLLS	94
HAWAIIAN SWEET BREAD	96
WHOLE WHEAT PUMPKIN BREAD	98
PUMPKIN BREAD WITH RAISINS AND PECANS	100
ORANGE PUMPKIN LOAF	102
DOWNEAST MAINE PUMPKIN BREAD	104
PUMPKIN CREAM CHEESE MUFFINS	106

INTRODUCTION

Nothing beats delicious, homemade bread! If you love homemade bread, you'll also love this book which contains delicious, easy, and unique bread-making recipes.

This book contains an ocean of delicious, tasty, quick, and Easy Bread recipes made with simple and readily available ingredients. Detailed instructions showing how to make bread and nutrition details are also added in the book!

So, let's first learn some basic things before jumping into the kitchen and prepare bread!

Main bread-making ingredient

The essential ingredient in the bread-making process is yeast. When preparing bread, you can use quick yeast and mix it with the rest of the dry ingredients right away. If you're using active dried yeast, dissolve it in warm water first before adding it to a recipe.

If your yeast is old or dead, your bread will not rise quickly. Keep your yeast in the refrigerator at all times to keep it fresh. In a small bowl, dissolve the yeast in warm water with a touch of sugar. If it isn't bubbly and frothy after ten minutes, toss it out and start over with fresh yeast.

After the yeast has risen to the surface, you'll combine a few additional basic ingredients to produce the dough.

At this point, it's important not to add too much flour. Adding the flour a bit at a time helps a lot. Add about half of the flour at a time until the dough achieves the desired consistency, then add the remaining flour 1/2 cup at a time until the dough reaches the desired consistency. It's simple to add more flour, but it's nearly impossible to undo when you've used too much. Allow the dough to rise for an hour before dividing it into two balls of similar size. Each dough ball should be rolled out into an eight-inch-long rectangle, then rolled up into a cylinder starting at the short edge. The texture and shape of the completed loaves are greatly improved by rolling the dough in this manner.

HOW LONG TO BAKE BREAD?

Bake for thirty to thirty-five minutes, or until golden brown and hollow when tapped on the bottom. After baking, brush the loaves with melted butter, but this is entirely optional. It softens the top crust slightly, and a little additional butter is never a bad thing, Right?

Allowing the bread to cool before slicing makes for smoother, more uniform slices.

The best bread pans

Pans made of aluminized steel or ceramic are the most popular. Both types of pans bake bread more uniformly and make it easier to remove the bread after baking. When using glass pans, it appears that your bread sinks too frequently, so it is not suggested. Also, dark or nonstick pans should be avoided because the bread would cook unevenly. It darkens on the outside before the inside of the bread is done, making it easier to cut.

Now, it's time to get ready and go into the kitchen. Let's go!

BASIC BABKA

Preparation: 30 Minutes

Cook: 35 Minutes

Servings: 24

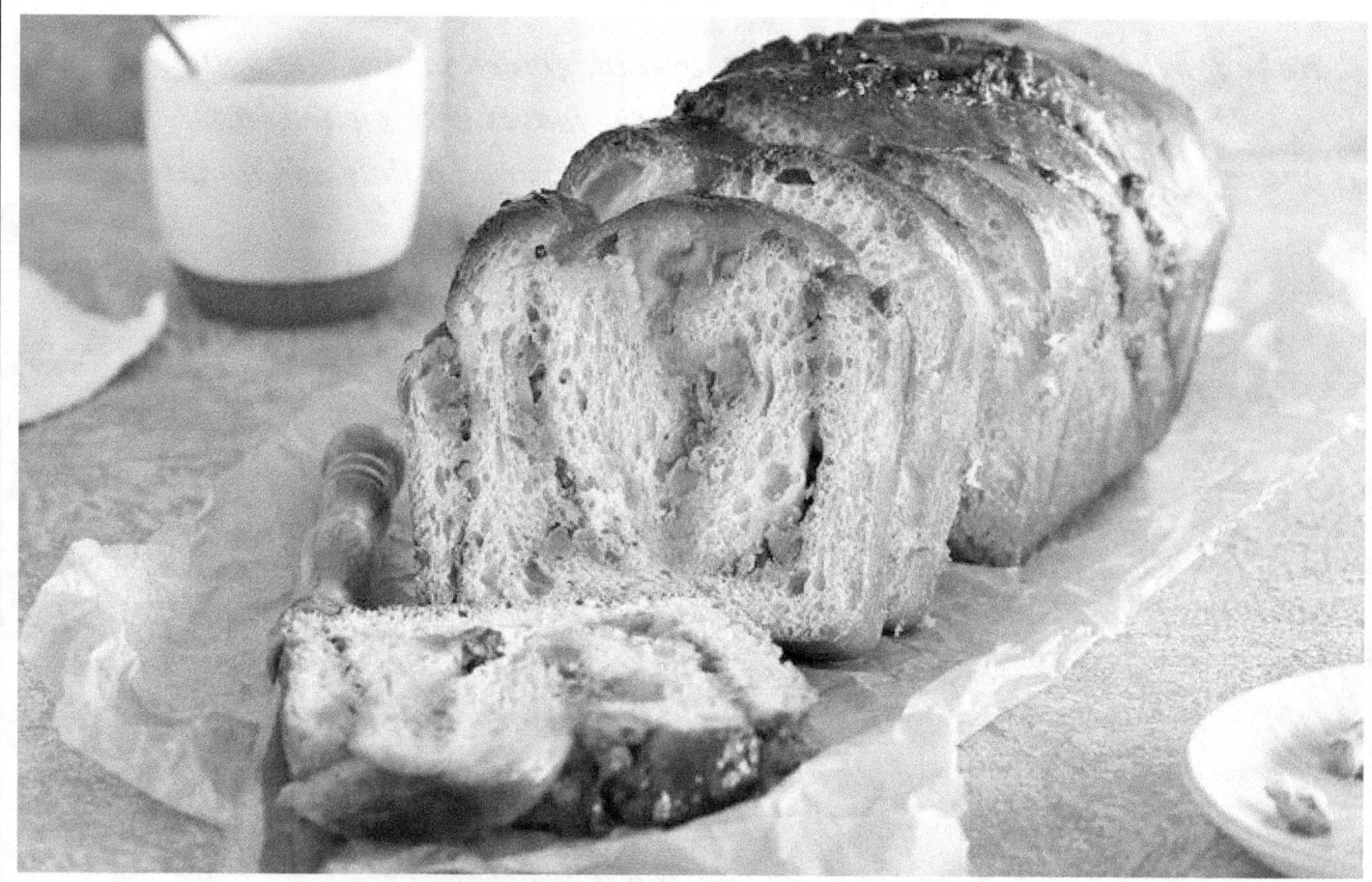

This sweet roll, swirl bread, and coffee cake hybrid is a Jewish delight. It's a sweet yeast dough that you roll out, stuff, and roll up like a jelly roll before cutting, twisting, and baking in a loaf pan. Don't worry: it may appear complicated, but it's actually rather simple. Once you've mastered the dough, you can experiment with different fillings.

Nutrition

Calories: 338 | Protein: 7.4g | Cholesterol: 54mg | Sodium: 158.1mg

Carbohydrates: 34.7g | Fat: 20g

Ingredients

For Dough

- 4 ½ cups all-purpose flour
- 2 eggs
- 1 cup hot milk (185 degrees F
- ½ cup white sugar)
- 2 packages active dry yeast
- ¼ cup butter
- 1 teaspoon salt
- ¼ cup warm water

For Walnut Filling

- 3 eggs
- 1 teaspoon vanilla extract
- 4 cups walnuts, chopped
- 1 ½ teaspoon ground cinnamon
- ⅓ cup butter, melted
- 2 tablespoons butter, melted
- 1 cup packed light brown sugar

Instructions

1. In a small bowl, whisk together the white sugar, 1/4 cup butter, and salt until the butter is melted and the mixture is lukewarm. Sprinkle yeast over warm water in the work bowl of a stand mixer fitted with a paddle; swirl to dissolve.
2. Combine the milk and yeast in a mixing bowl. 2 eggs and 2 1/2 cups flour; beat on high until thoroughly mixed. Add the remaining 2 cups flour, 1/2 cup at a time, to the mixer on low speed.
3. Place dough in a large lightly greased mixing basin and turn to coat the surface. Switch to the dough hook and mix for five minutes, or until the dough leaves the sides of the bowl. Cover with a cloth and set aside to rise until doubled in size, about one hour.
4. While the dough rises, prepare the walnut filling. In a large mixing bowl, lightly beat 3 eggs. Brown sugar, 1/3 cup melted butter, cinnamon, and vanilla essence are added to the mixture. Toss in the walnuts.

5. Knead the dough. Turn out the dough onto a large, lightly floured surface, cover, and set aside for ten minutes. By using parchment paper, line three 9x5-inch loaf pans, leaving a 2-inch overhang on long sides.
6. On a lightly floured board, divide the dough into thirds and roll each third out to a 12-inch square.
7. Fill each dough square with 1/3 of the walnut filling and distribute to within 1/2 inch of the edges. As if you were making a jelly roll, roll each piece tightly. To seal the ends and seams, pinch them together. Roll logs back and forth with your palms until they are equally round.
8. Cut 1 log in half lengthwise with a sharp knife or dough scraper to make 2 striped strands. Twist strands loosely together with cut sides facing out in 2 or 3 wide, horizontal twists, working fast. Fit into one of the prepared pans, tucking any loose filling beneath and patting back any slack filling. It may appear to be a chaos right now, but it turns out nicely.
9. Rep with the rest of the logs and pans. Cover pans with a towel and place in a warm place to rise for one hour or until doubled in size. The tops of the loaves should not rise above the pans' top edges.
10. Preheat the oven to 350 degrees Fahrenheit. Brush the remaining 2 tablespoons of melted butter over the tops of the loaves.
11. 35 to 45 minutes until loaves are puffy and thoroughly browned, and a thermometer inserted in the center registers 200 degrees F. If the tops of the loaves start to brown before they're done, cover them with foil. Cool for ten minutes in the pans before removing with paper and transferring to a wire rack. Allow one hour to cool completely. If desired, glaze before slicing crosswise to serve.

SWEET CHALLAH BREAD

Preparation: 1 Hour

Cook: 30 Minutes

Servings: 20

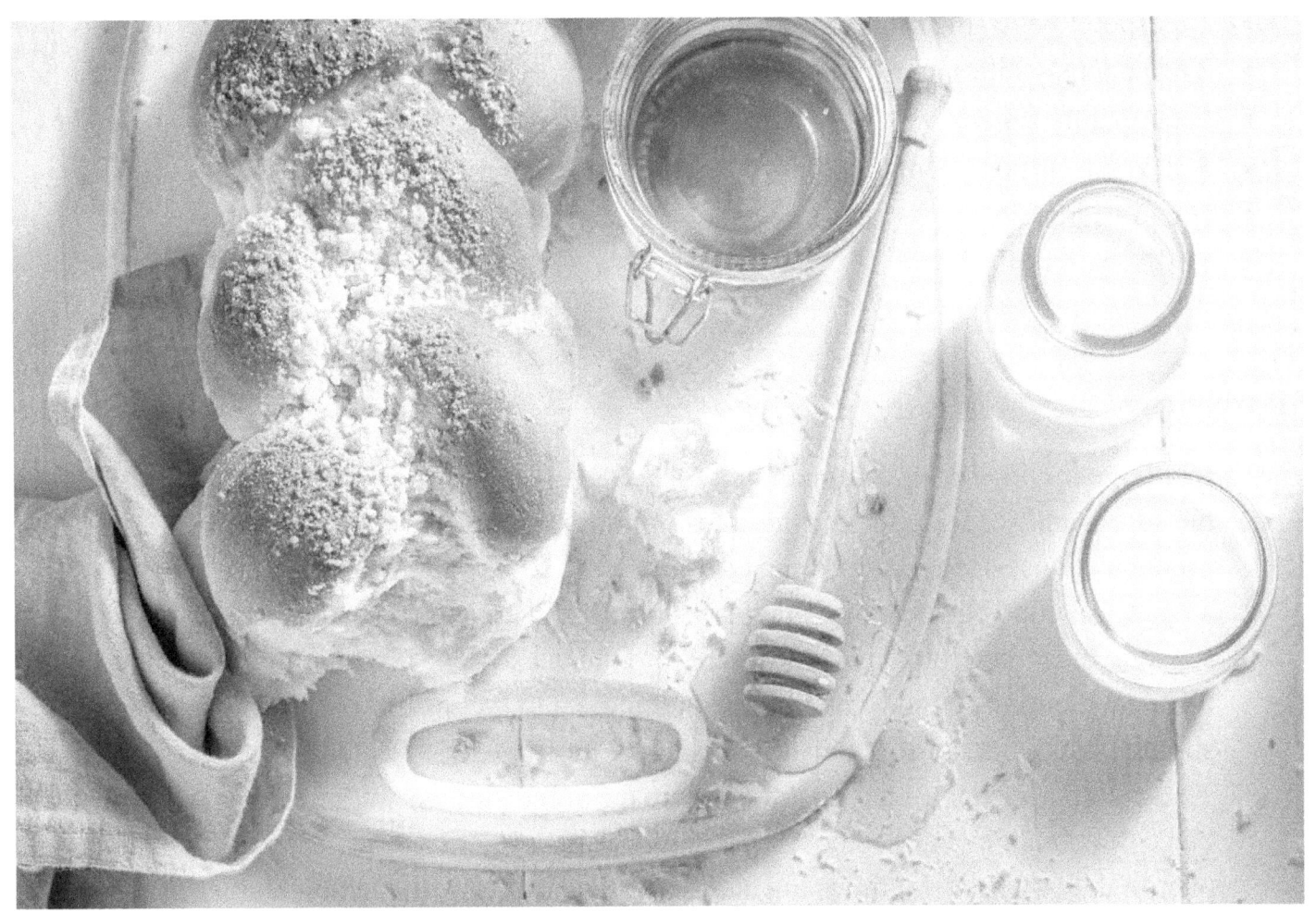

This is a delicious bread that comes together quickly. It's so excellent that a 30-year-old man who ate it at my Shabbat Table laughed out loud. The bread should be baked for a shorter time if you want it to be doughier.

Nutrition

Calories: 328 | Protein: 7.6g | Cholesterol: 46.5mg | Sodium: 368.5mg

Carbohydrates: 57g | Fat: 7.5g

Ingredients

- 4 eggs
- 1 egg
- 1 teaspoon water
- 1 cup white sugar
- 2 cups warm water
- 6 cups all-purpose flour, or as needed
- 1 tablespoon active dry yeast
- 1 teaspoon vegetable oil
- 2 teaspoons white sugar
- ⅓ cup white sugar
- 3 cups all-purpose flour
- ½ cup vegetable oil
- 1 tablespoon salt

Instructions

1. In a large mixing bowl, combine the yeast, 1/3 cup sugar, and warm water, stir to dissolve the sugar, and set aside for five minutes or until a creamy layer develops on top. To produce a loose sponge, add 3 cups of flour.
2. 4 eggs, 1/2 cup vegetable oil, 1 tablespoon salt, and 1 cup sugar, whisked together in a separate dish, then fold the egg mixture into the yeast-flour mixture until thoroughly blended. Continue to add flour 1 cup at a time, up to 9 cups total. The dough should be slightly sticky but not soggy that it sticks to your fingers.
3. To develop gluten, turn the dough out onto a floured surface and knead for five minutes. Place the dough in an oiled bowl and shape it into a tight spherical shape. Turn the dough over in the bowl several times to coat the surface, cover with a cloth, and let rise in a warm environment until doubled in size, about one hour. Punch down the dough and knead for five minutes more, or until smooth and elastic.
4. Line baking pans with parchment paper or grease them. In a small bowl, whisk together 1 egg, 1 teaspoon oil, 2 teaspoons sugar, and 1 teaspoon water. Refrigerate until ready to use. To make a 3-strand braided loaf, divide the dough into four parts and cut each piece into three smaller pieces. Roll the little dough pieces into ropes about the thickness of your thumb and about 12 inches long on a floured surface. The center of the rope should be thicker than the ends, and the ends should be thinner. Braid three ropes at the top by pinching them together. Begin with the strand on the right and work your way to the left,

passing over the middle strand (that strand becomes the new middle strand.) Move the strand that is furthest to the left over the new middle strand.
5. Continue braiding until the loaf is braided, alternating sides each time, and squeeze the ends together and fold them underneath for a clean look. Location the loaves on the prepared baking sheets and let rise in a warm place for thirty to forty-five minutes, or until doubled in size. Brush a thin layer of egg glaze over the tops of the bread and set aside the rest.
6. Preheat the oven to 350 degrees Fahrenheit
7. Bake the bread for twenty minutes in a preheated oven, then take it from the oven and brush the bread with a second layer of glaze. Return to the oven and bake for another five to ten minutes, or until the tops are beautiful and golden brown. Allow it to cool completely before cutting.

IRRESISTIBLE WHOLE WHEAT CHALLAH

Preparation: 30 Minutes

Cook: 30 Minutes

Servings: 16

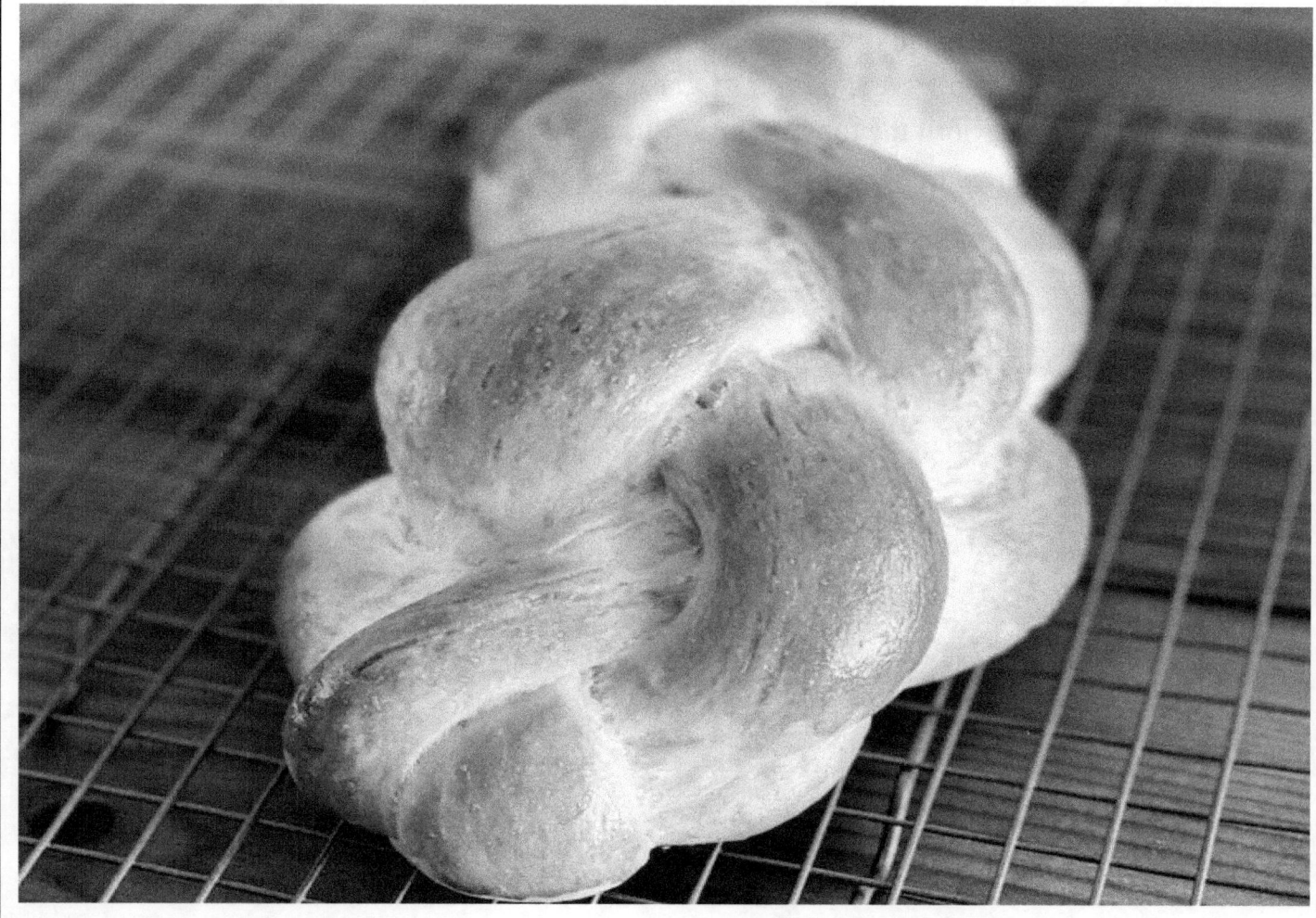

It's a fantastic present or dessert for any occasion, warm and light right out of the oven with butter and salt sprinkled on top. It's best to use whole wheat flour, although white flour or a combination of the two would suffice. It's simple and enjoyable, but it takes all day. It's really worth it, believe me

Nutrition Facts

Calories: 215 | Protein: 5.8g | Cholesterol: 23.3mg | Sodium: 157.1mg

Carbohydrates: 32.9g | Fat: 8g

Ingredients

- 2 eggs
- 1 cup warm water
- 2 ¼ teaspoons active dry yeast
- ½ cup honey
- ½ cup olive oil
- 4 cups whole wheat flour
- 1 teaspoon salt
- ¼ cup raisins, to taste (Optional)
- 2 tablespoons vital wheat gluten (optional)

Instructions

1. Combine the flour, salt, yeast, and vital wheat gluten in a large mixing bowl and stir thoroughly. Mix the honey, olive oil, water, eggs, and raisins in a separate bowl. Pour the liquid mixture into the flour mixture, constantly stirring until a dough form.
2. Turn the dough out onto a floured surface and knead for ten minutes, or until smooth and elastic. Make a circle out of the dough. Place the dough in a dish that has been lightly oiled. And turn the dough over a few times to grease the surface. Cover the bowl with a cloth and set it aside to rise for one hour in a warm, draft-free place.
3. Punch down the dough, knead it a few times to eliminate some of the air bubbles, then cut it into two pieces of similar size. While shaping or braiding the first loaf, place 1 piece of dough beneath a damp cloth to keep it from drying out.
4. Roll the little dough pieces into ropes about the thickness of your thumb and about 12 inches long on a floured surface. The center of the rope should be thicker than the ends, and the ends should be thinner. Braid three ropes at the top by pinching them together. Begin with the strand on the right and work your way to the left, passing over the middle strand becomes the new middle strand.
5. Move the strand that is furthest to the left over the new middle strand. Continue braiding until the loaf is braided, alternating sides each time, and squeeze the ends together and fold them underneath for a clean look. Repeat with the remaining loaf, then set the braided loaves on a baking sheet lined with parchment paper and let rise until doubled, about thirty minutes.
6. Preheat the oven to 350 degrees Fahrenheit. Bake for thirty minutes in a preheated oven until golden brown. For the finest flavor, serve warm.

MOST AMAZING CHALLAH

Preparation: 40 Minutes

Cook: 30 Minutes

Servings: 32

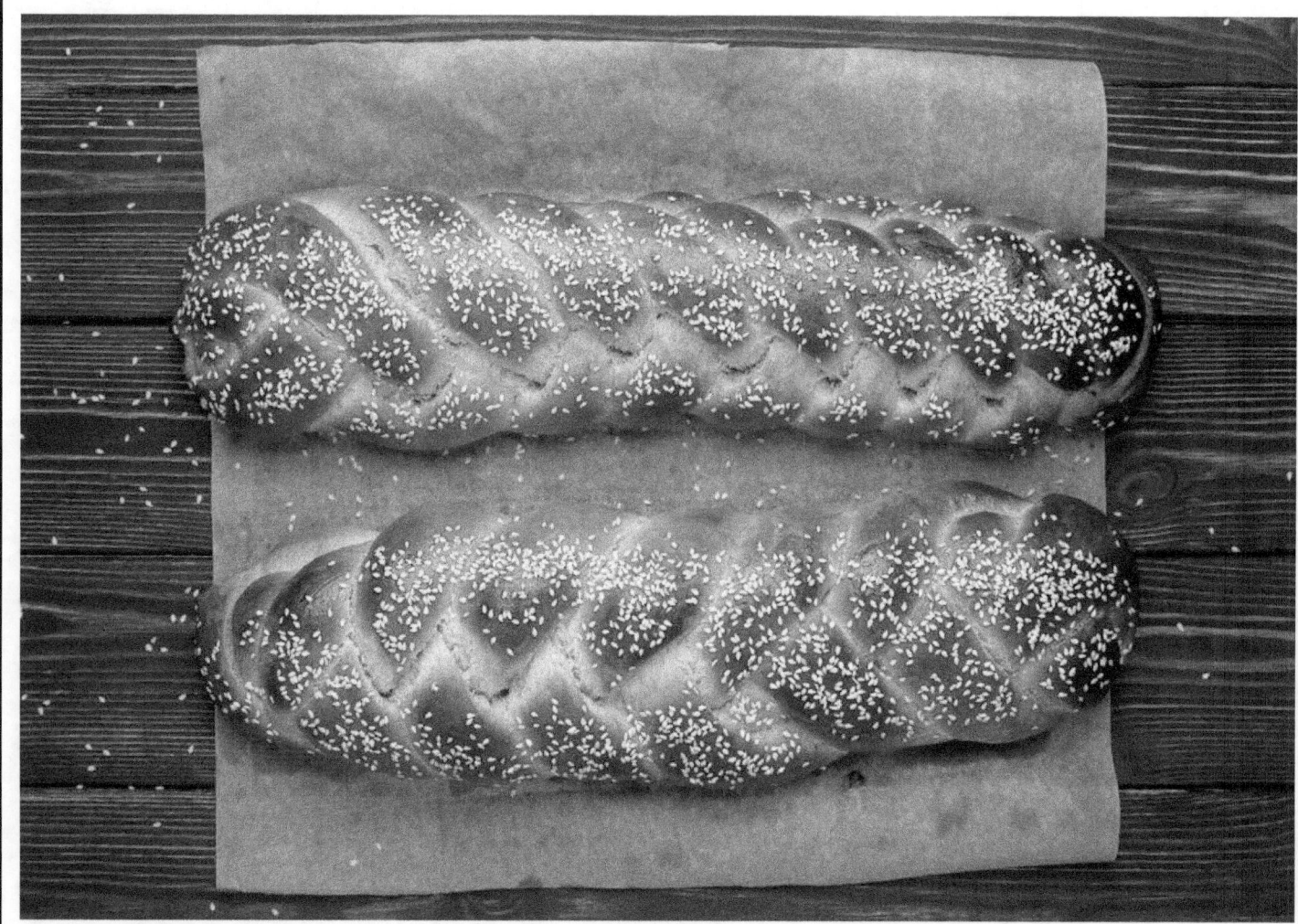

We made my own Challah, which turned out to be fantastic! It takes advantage of rapid-rise yeast, which saves you a lot of time. Enjoy! We tried a lot of different combinations before we got it right.

Nutrition

Calories: 274 | Protein: 7.7g | Cholesterol: 29.1mg | Sodium: 515.2mg

Carbohydrates: 42.7g | Fat: 7.8g

Ingredients

- 4 eggs
- 2 tablespoons salt
- ¾ cup white sugar
- 1 cup pareve margarine, melted
- 12 cups bread flour, or as needed
- 1 egg 4 packages quick-rise yeast
- 4 cups warm water
- ¼ cup sesame seeds, divided
- ½ teaspoon vanilla extract

Instructions

1. In a large mixing bowl, sprinkle the yeast over the water and gently stir to hydrate the yeast. Mix in the salt, sugar, margarine, and 4 eggs until thoroughly combined. Gradually add the flour, up to 12 cups at a time, until the dough is somewhat sticky but not moist. Knead the dough on a floured surface for eight to ten minutes. Set aside baking sheets that have been greased or lined with parchment paper. s, or until smooth and elastic.
2. Cut the bread dough into four pieces of similar size. For 3-strand braided bread, cut each piece into thirds. Roll the little dough pieces into ropes about the thickness of your thumb and about 12 inches long on a floured surface. The center of the rope should be thicker than the ends, and the ends should be thinner. Braid three ropes at the top by pinching them together. Begin with the strand on the right and work your way to the left, passing over the middle strand. Move the strand that is furthest to the left over the new middle strand. Continue braiding until the loaf is braided, alternating sides each time, and squeeze the ends together and fold them underneath for a clean look. Carry on with the remaining loaves in the same manner. Place the loaves on the prepared baking sheets and let rise for one to one and half hours, or until doubled in size.
Preheat the oven to 350 degrees Fahrenheit. Whisk 1 egg with vanilla extract in a small bowl, and brush the loaves with the egg wash. Sprinkle each loaf with about 1 tablespoon of sesame seeds.
3. Bake for thirty minutes in a preheated oven until the tops are beautiful and golden brown. Allow it to cool completely before slicing.

MIRIAM'S NOT-SO-SECRET CHALLAH

Preparation: 30 Minutes

Cook: 45 Minutes

Servings: 20

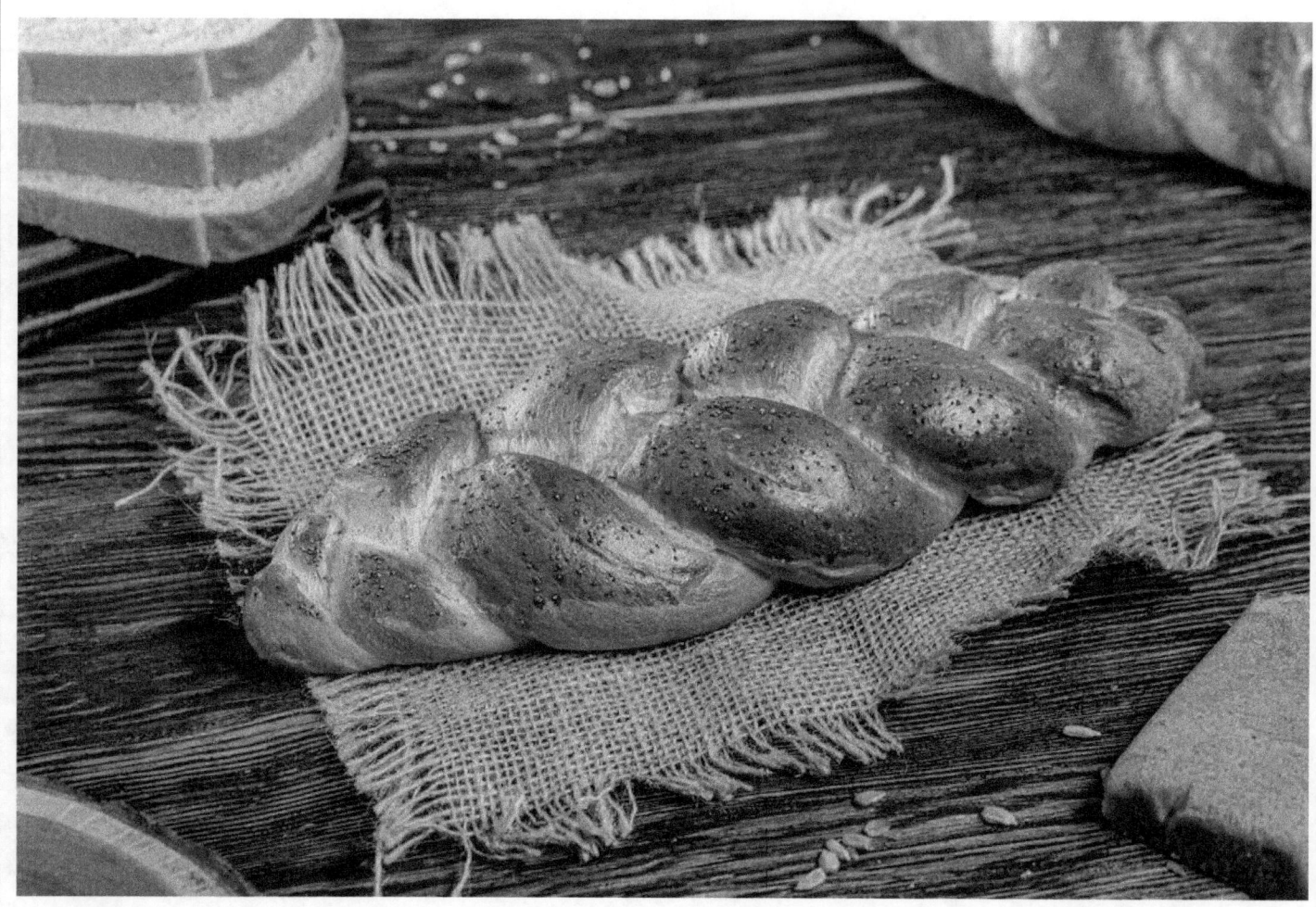

A delightfully sweet yet light challah that adds a distinctive touch to every evening. If you want, you can knead some raisins into the dough.

Nutrition

Calories: 253 | Protein: 7.8g | Cholesterol: 46.5mg | Sodium: 421.7mg

Carbohydrates: 39.7g | Fat: 6.8g

Ingredients

- 4 eggs
- 3 packages active dry yeast
- 2 cups water
- ½ cup margarine
- ¼ cup white sugar
- ¼ cup brown sugar
- 7 cups bread flour, divided
- 1 tablespoon salt
- 1 egg, beaten
- 1 tablespoon poppy seeds

Instructions

1. Water and margarine will be combined in a small saucepan. Heat until the margarine is completely melted and the mixture is quite warm but not boiling.
2. Combine 3 cups flour, white sugar, brown sugar, yeast, and salt in a large mixing bowl. Mix in the water and margarine mixture thoroughly. One at a time, add 4 eggs, beating well after each addition. 1/2 cup at a time, add the remaining flour, mixing well after each addition. Turn the dough out onto a lightly floured area and knead for about eight minutes, or until smooth and elastic. Lightly grease a large mixing bowl, then set the dough in it and turn to coat it in oil. Cover with a moist towel and set aside in a warm place to rise for one hour or until doubled in volume. Form the dough into long 'ropes' by dividing it into six equal pieces. To make two huge loaves, braid the pieces together. Place the loaves on two lightly oiled cookie sheets, cover with a damp cloth, and let rise for about forty minutes, or until doubled in volume. Preheat the oven to 350 degrees Fahrenheit
3. Brush the poppy seeds on the risen loaves and brush them with the beaten egg. Bake for forty-five minutes in a preheated oven or until the bread sounds hollow when tapped.

SY'S CHALLAH

Preparation: 30 Minutes

Cook: 45 Minutes

Servings: 24

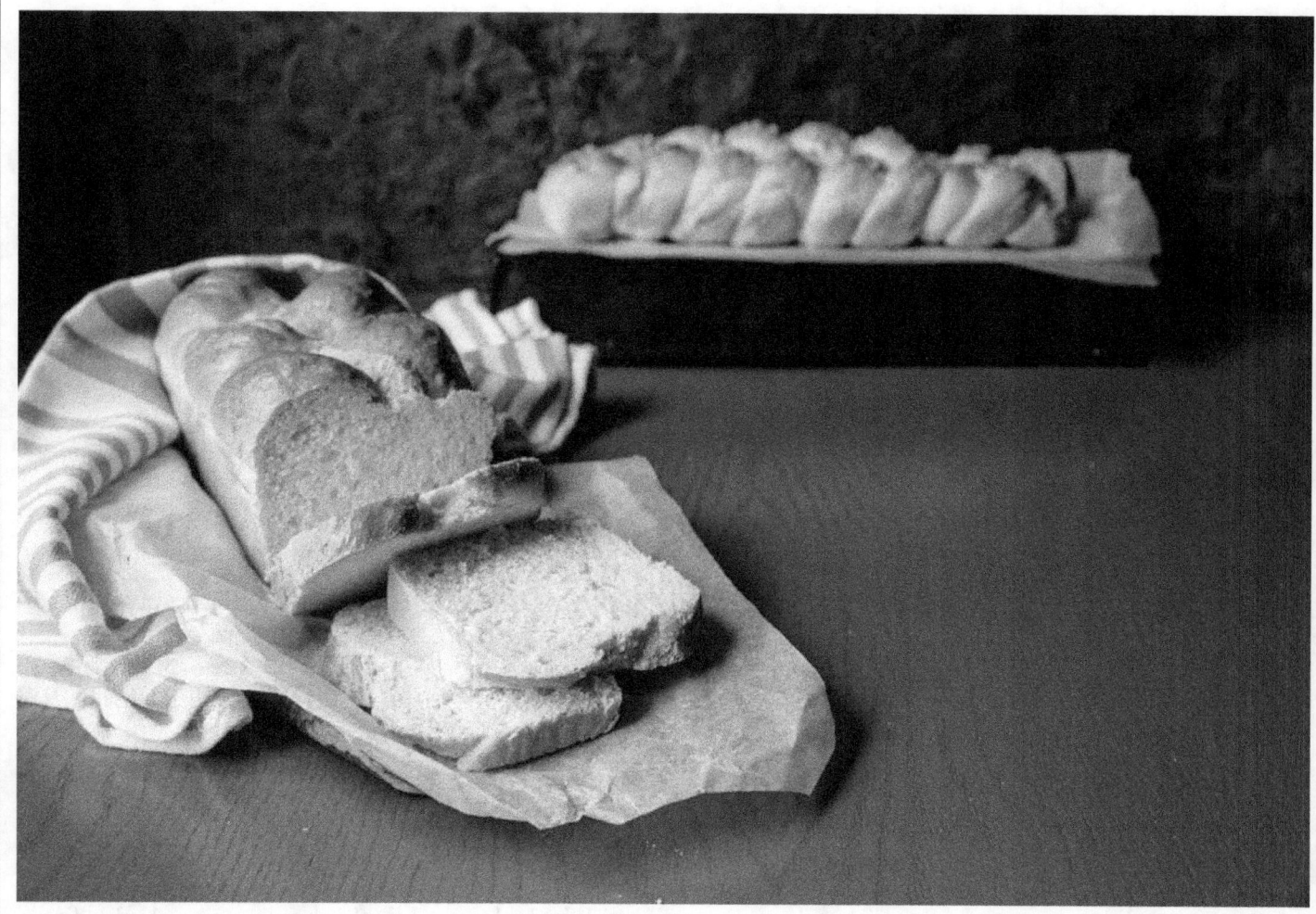

An almost fail-proof recipe designed for optimal flavor and ease of preparation. If you want to make it sweeter, use 1/2 cup sugar instead of 1/4 cup.

Nutrition

Calories: 158 | Protein: 4.6g | Cholesterol: 31mg | Sodium: 303.3mg

Carbohydrates: 26.3g | Fat: 3.6g

Ingredients

- 1 egg
- 3 eggs
- 6 cups all-purpose flour
- 2 packages of active dry yeast
- ¼ cup white sugar
- 1 tablespoon salt
- ¼ cup vegetable oil
- 1 ¼ cups warm water
- 1 tablespoon poppy seeds (optional)

Instructions

1. In a large mixing bowl or a mixing bowl for an electric mixer with a dough hook, combine the sugar, salt, and oil. Stir in boiling water to dissolve the sugar and salt. Stir in the yeast and set aside until the mixture foams up. Pour in the lightly beaten eggs. Add 4 1/2 cups flour to the yeast mixture if using an electric mixer. Mix until all of the flour is included, and the dough becomes stringy. This stringiness implies the presence of gluten. Continue to add flour until the dough hook completely covers the dough; 1 or 2 cups is generally plenty. Allow the hook to knead for several minutes. The dough should be elastic and silky. Stir 4 1/2 cups flour into the yeast mixture to knead by hand. Work 1 to 2 cups of flour into the soft dough on a lightly floured surface. Knead for eight to ten minutes, or until smooth and elastic.
2. Place dough in a greased mixing bowl and turn to coat the surface. Using a moist cloth, cover the bowl. Allow dough to rise until it has doubled in size. After the first rise, punch down and allow to rise again. The first rising takes approximately one hour, while the second takes forty-five minutes. A nicer bread comes from two risings, but if time is an issue, just do one.
3. Divide the dough in half and then into three or four equal halves. Make two braids with the bread and set them on a greased baking sheet. Allow rising until twice in size. Using a beaten egg, brush the surface. If desired, top with poppy seeds.
4. Preheat oven to 350°F and bake for thirty-five minutes, or until golden brown. Place the loaves on a wire rack to cool.

SHABBAT CHALLAH

Preparation: 45 Minutes

Cook: 45 Minutes

Servings: 60

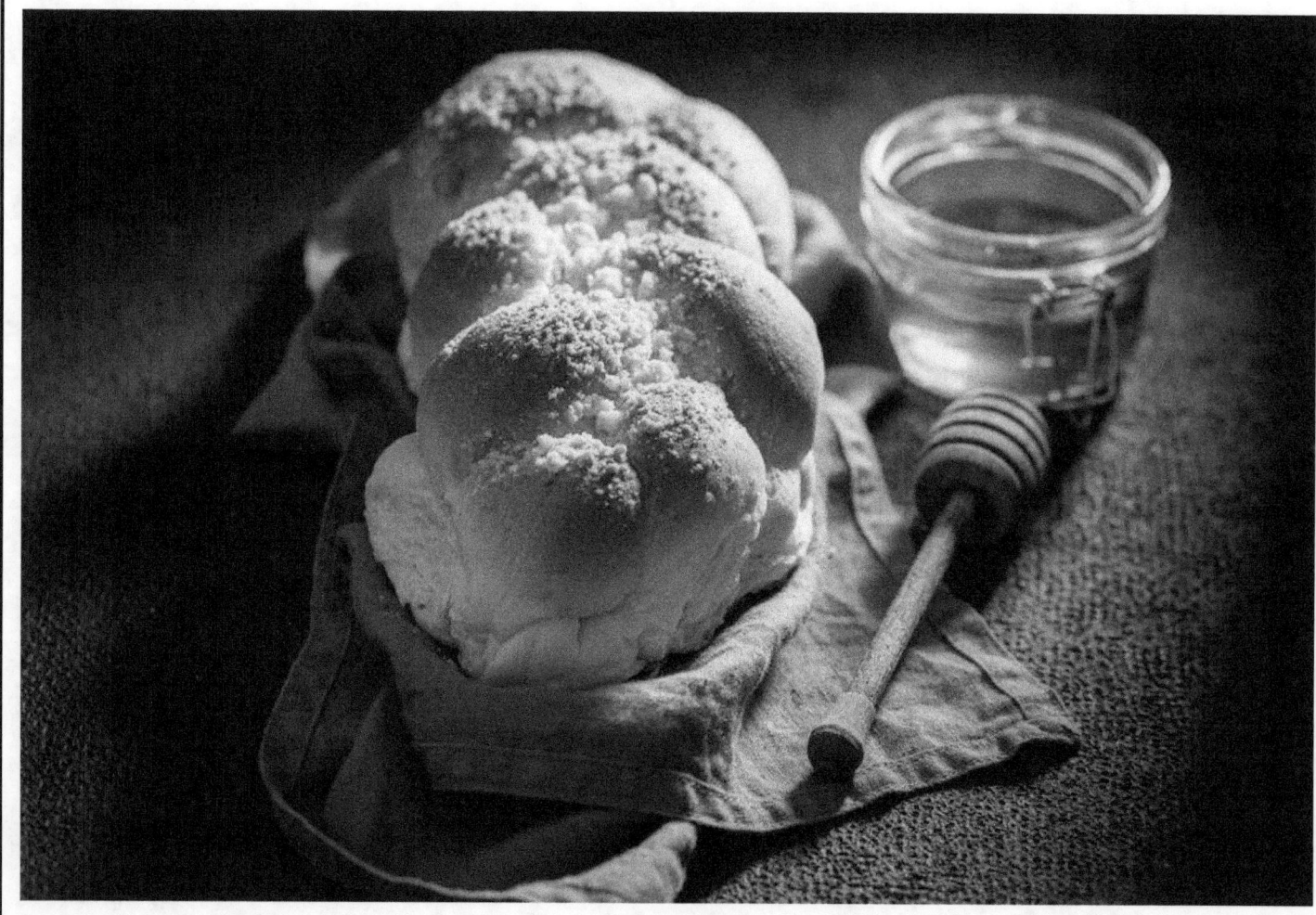

My Shabbat Challah is amazing. We made it up on the spot because we didn't like the ones we tried. You will enjoy it if you give it a try!! This recipe yields 6 standard loaves or two big braided loaves.

Nutrition

Calories: 168 | Protein: 3.4g | Cholesterol: 15.5mg | Sodium: 239.7mg

Carbohydrates: 21.2g | Fat: 4.6g

Ingredients

- 4 eggs
- 1 egg
- 2 tablespoons salt
- ½ cup white sugar
- 12 cups all-purpose flour
- 3 tablespoons water
- 4 cups warm water
- ½ teaspoon vanilla sugar, or vanilla extract 1 cup vegetable oil
- 3 tablespoons active dry yeast
- ¼ cup sesame seeds

Instructions

1. Sprinkle the yeast over the water in a large mixing bowl. Allow for about five minutes for the yeast to dissolve. Stir in the salt, sugar, oil, and four eggs until everything is well combined. Gradually incorporate the flour. Turn the dough out onto a floured surface and knead for eight to ten minutes when it gets too stiff to stir. Place the dough underneath the bowl to rise until it has doubled in size. Alternatively, you can put the dough in a bowl and cover it with a towel.
2. Depending on the form you want, punch down the dough and divide it into 6 or 8 even pieces. Remember to remove a little bit and bless it. Make ropes out of the parts. Braid into two loaves or one giant 6-piece braid if your oven is large enough. Alternatively, each rope can be used to form spiral challahs. Tuck the ends under and place on a baking pan to rise until a small depression is left in the bread when lightly poked. Preheat oven to 400 degrees Fahrenheit (200 degrees C). Combine the remaining egg, water, and vanilla sugar in a mixing bowl. Brush the tops of the loaves with a brush. Sesame seeds can be sprinkled on top.
3. Preheat the oven to 350°F and bake the bread for thirty-five to forty minutes, or until golden brown. While the other loaves are baking, wrap the tiny piece of dough blessed in aluminum foil and burn it as an offering in the oven.

MICHELL JENNY'S CHALLAH

Preparation: 40 Minutes

Cook: 30 Minutes

Servings: 32

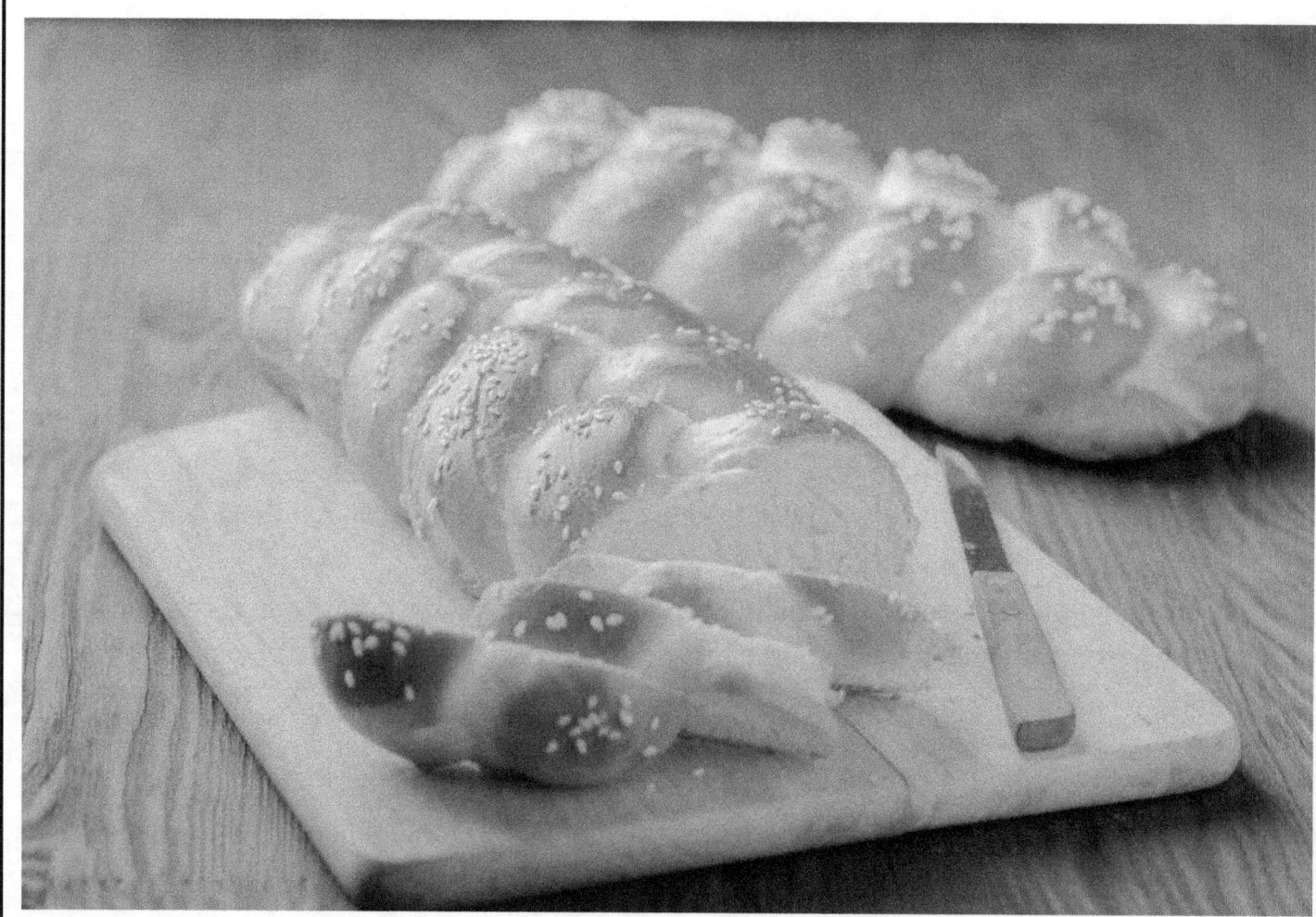

This is a household favorite. My dearest buddy gave me the recipe as a gift.

Nutrition

Calories: 193 | Protein: 4.3g | Fat: 5.5g | Cholesterol: 7.8mg

Sodium: 626.1mg | Carbohydrates: 31.7g

Ingredients

- 2 eggs
- 4 cups all-purpose flour
- 2 teaspoons active dry yeast
- ⅞ cup water
- ½ tablespoon salt
- ¼ cup honey
- ¼ cup butter, melted

Instructions

1. In the bread machine, combine the water, salt, honey, eggs, melted butter or margarine, flour, and yeast in the order listed. Start the machine on the Dough cycle.
2. After the dough has initially risen, remove it from the machine. Make three or four equal pieces of dough. Braid the pieces together and tuck the ends under to seal them. Place on a baking tray that has been buttered. This bread can also be baked in a prepared 9 x 5-inch loaf pan. Allow the dough to rise until it has doubled in size.
3. Preheat the oven to 350 degrees Fahrenheit
4. Bake for thirty-five to forty-five minutes in a preheated oven until the crust is a rich golden color.

EKMEK TURKISH BREAD

Preparation: 1 Hour

Cook: 40 Minutes

Servings: 12

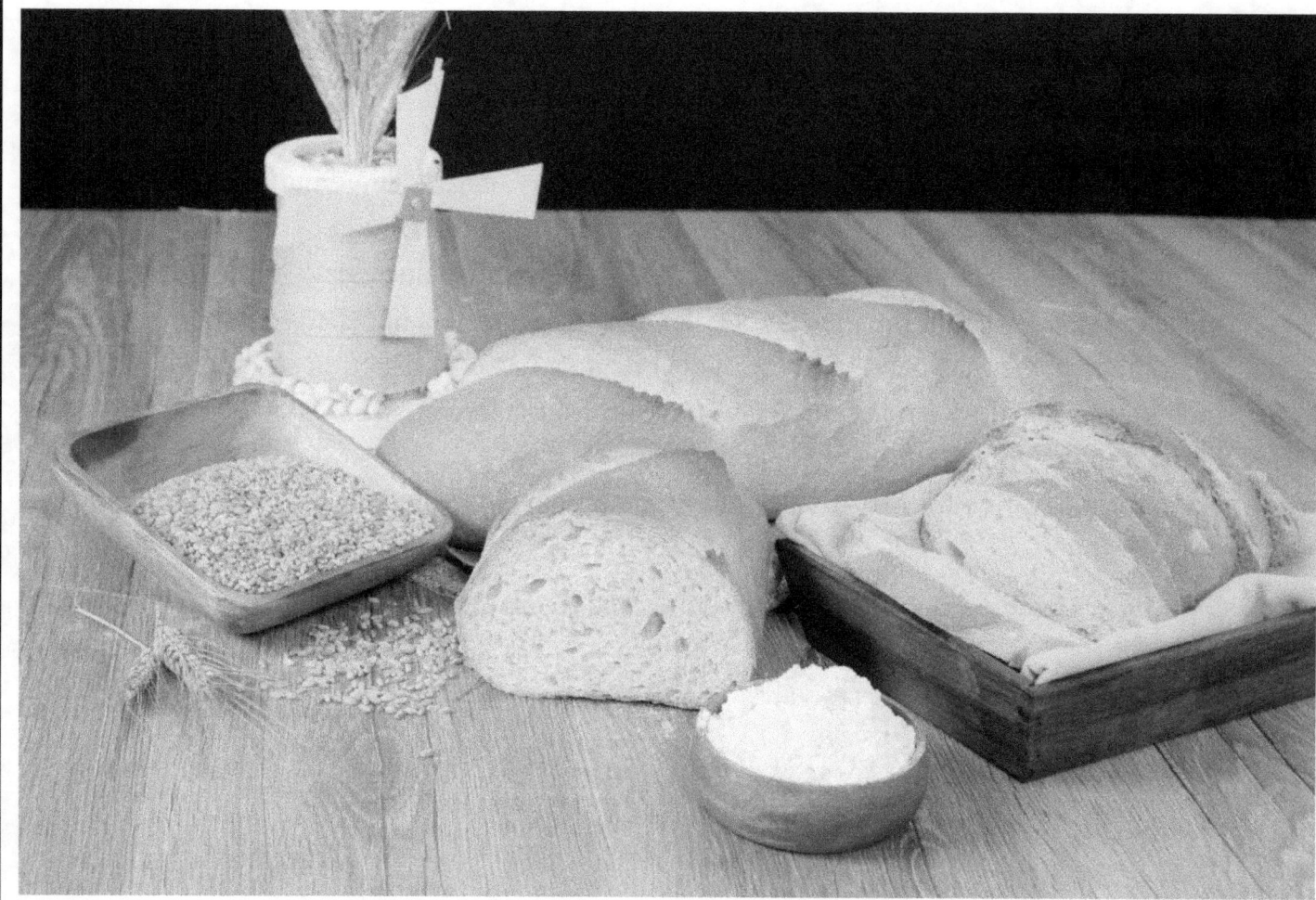

Ekmek is a light, slightly tangy flatbread that pairs well with Havarti. It starts with a starter that ferments for four days. We recommend baking the loaves on a pizza stone. If you don't have a pizza stone, cookie sheets will suffice. The recipe appears to be difficult, but it is simpler than it appears.

Nutrition

Calories: 6 | Fat: 0.1g | Sodium: 390mg | Protein: 0.6g | Carbohydrates: 1g

Ingredients

- 6 cups bread flour
- 5 teaspoons active dry yeast
- 2 cups warm water
- 1 teaspoon white sugar
- 1 ½ cups bread flour, divided
- ¾ cup water, divided
- 2 teaspoons salt

Instructions

1. To make the starter, follow these steps: In a coverable bowl, combine 1/2 cup flour and 1/4 cup water and whisk thoroughly. Allow to sit at room temperature overnight, covered. Add 1/2 cup flour and 1/4 cup water to the bowl the next day. Allow to sit at room temperature overnight, covered. Add 1/2 cup flour and 1/4 cup water to the bowl on the third day. Allow to sit at room temperature overnight, covered.
2. To make the dough: Dissolve the yeast and sugar in the warm water in a large mixing basin. Allow ten minutes for the mixture to become creamy.
3. Add the starter to the yeast mixture after breaking it up into small pieces. Combine 4 cups of flour and salt in a mixing bowl. 1/2 cup at a time, add the remaining flour, beating well after each addition. When the dough has come together, turn it out onto a lightly floured surface and knead for about eight minutes, or until smooth and elastic. Cover the dough with a dry cloth after sprinkling it with flour. Let it rise until double in size.
4. Return the dough to a lightly floured work surface and deflate it. Divide the dough in half and knead for two to three minutes on each half. Make a compact oval loaf out of each piece. Sprinkle two sheet pans with cornmeal. Two loaves will be rolled and stretched into 15x12 inch ovals. Using flour, lightly dust the tops of the loaves. Allow rising in a warm area until doubled in size, covered with a dry cloth. Preheat the oven to 425 degrees F in the meantime.
5. Preheat the oven to 350°F and bake for thirty to forty minutes. In the first fifteen minutes, mist three times with water. When you tap the bottom of a loaf, this will sound hollow. Allow it to cool completely on wire racks before serving.

SYRIAN BREAD

Preparation: 20 Minutes

Cook: 10 Minutes

Servings: 8

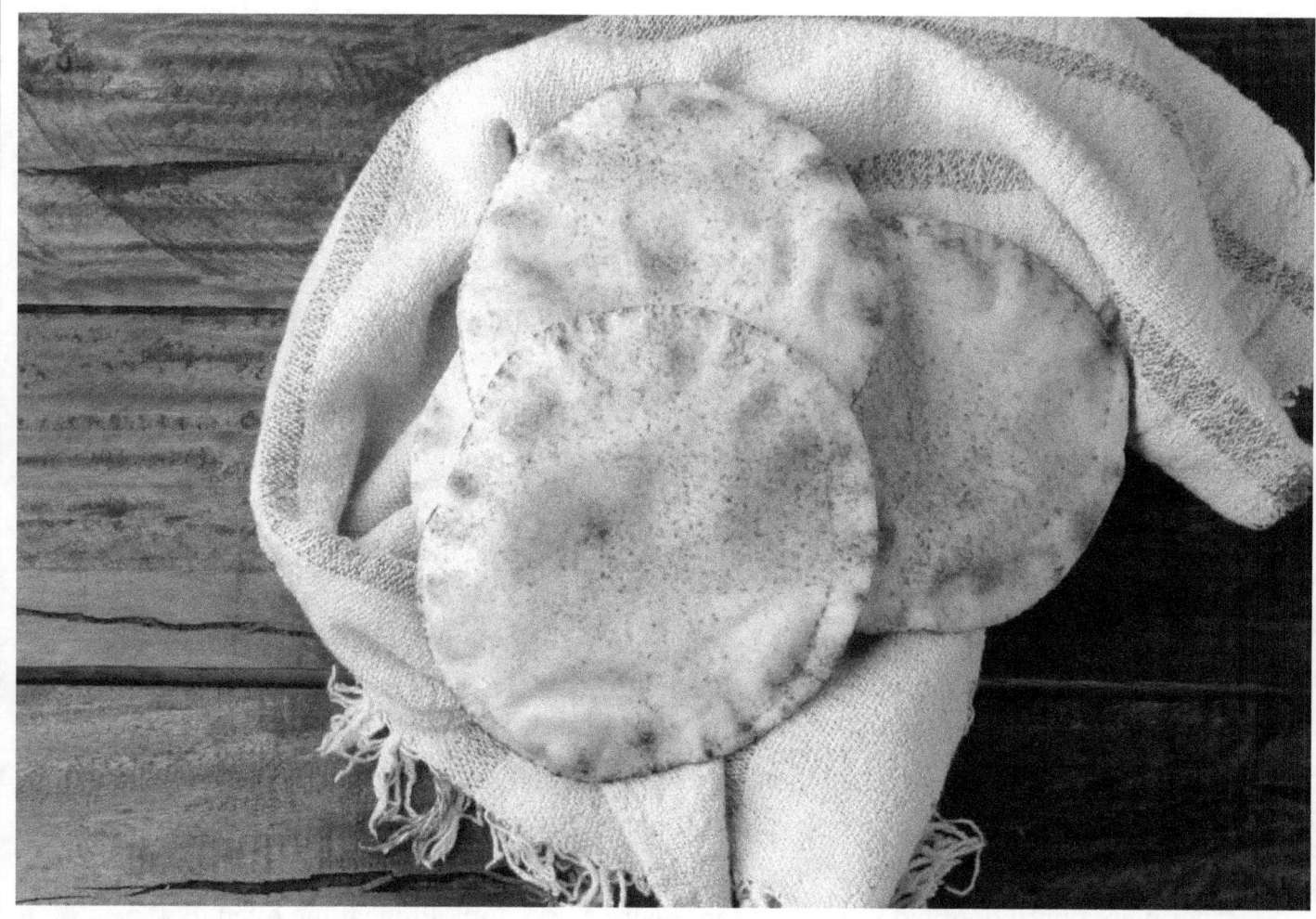

Bake the dough in the oven after mixing it in your bread machine. This is a versatile Middle Eastern flatbread that can be served for lunch or dinner.

Nutrition

Calories: 204 | Protein: 5.1g | Fat: 3.9g | Sodium: 438.3mg | Carbohydrates: 36.3g

Ingredients

- 3 cups all-purpose flour
- ½ teaspoon white sugar
- 1 ½ teaspoon active dry yeast
- 1.063 cups water
- 2 tablespoons vegetable oil
- 1 ½ teaspoons salt

Instructions

1. Place the ingredients in the bread machine pan in the manufacturer's recommended order. Select the Dough cycle and push the Start button.
2. Preheat the oven to 475 degrees Fahrenheit
3. Turn the dough out onto a lightly floured surface once it has risen. Form the dough into rounds by dividing it into eight equal pieces. Allow the rounds to rest by covering them with a moist cloth. Make thin, flat rings out of the dough, about 8 inches in diameter. Cook two at a time on hot baking sheets or a baking stone for about five minutes, or until puffed up and golden brown. Continue with the remaining loaves.

SERENDIPITY BREAD

Preparation: 15 Minutes

Cook: 15 Minutes

Servings: 10

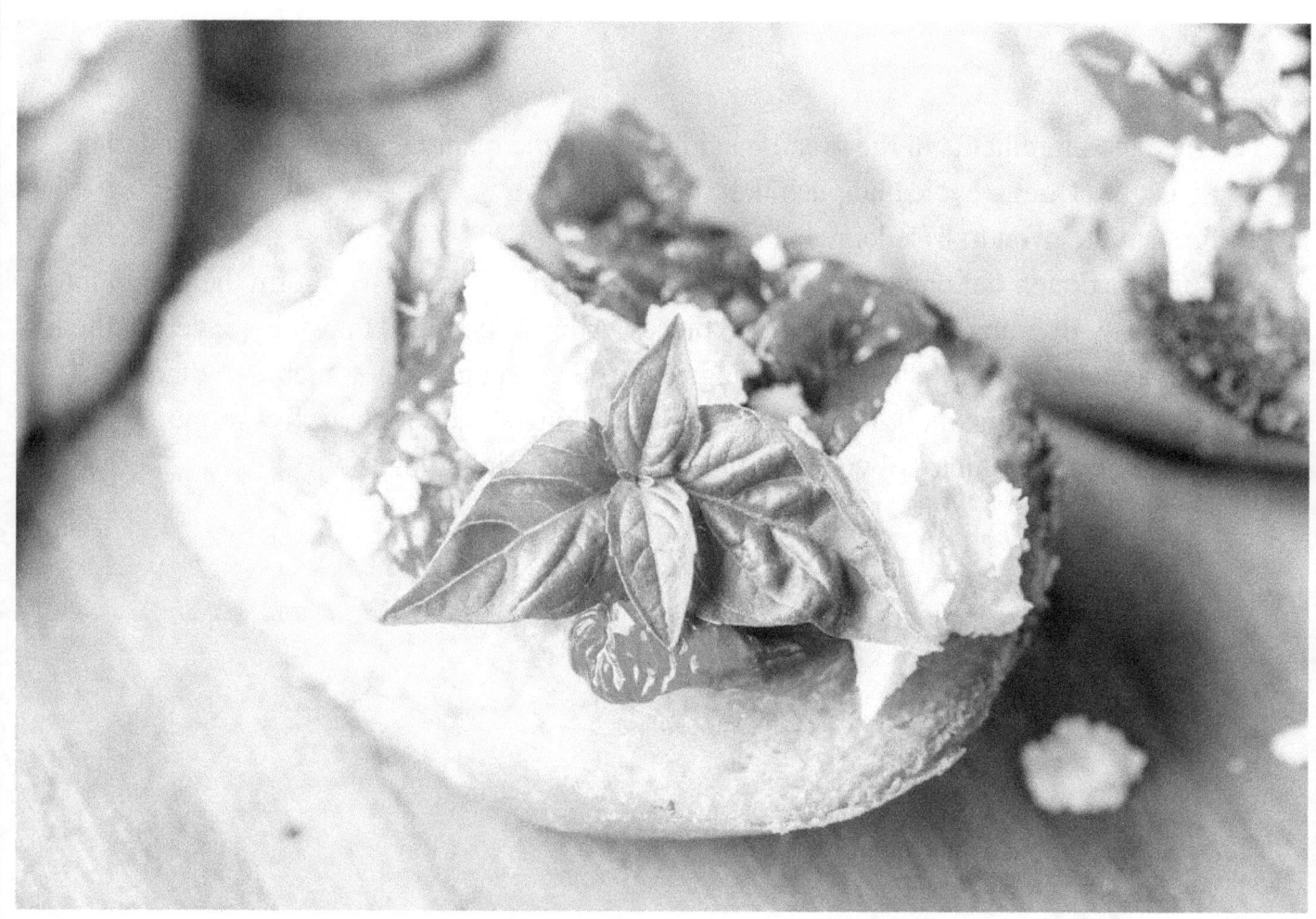

A flatbread made in a bread machine and finished on an outside grill. When the power went out for the entire day, my sister had a batch of bread dough rising in her bread machine when she 'found' this bread. Incredible.

Nutrition

Calories: 93 | Protein: 2.5g | Cholesterol: 16.5mg | Sodium: 501mg

Carbohydrates: 4.4g | Fat: 7.5g

Ingredients

- 2 tablespoons olive oil
- 3 ⅓ cups bread flour
- 1 ½ teaspoon active dry yeast
- 1 ½ teaspoons salt
- 1 ¼ cups water
- 2 tablespoons butter
- 2 tablespoons milk powder
- 2 tablespoons white sugar
- 2 teaspoons garlic powder (Optional)
- 4 ounces crumbled feta cheese (Optional)

Instructions

1. Place the first set of ingredients in the bread machine pan in the manufacturer's recommended order. Select the DOUGH cycle and press the START button. Remove the olive oil, garlic powder, and feta cheese from the mix.
2. Preheat a medium-hot outside grill. Turn the dough out onto a lightly floured surface and divide it into two pieces when the cycle is finished. Each half will be rolled out into a 9- to 10-inch-wide circle. Apply olive oil to the tops of each round.
3. Place the bread circles on the grill with the oil side down. Brush the opposite side with olive oil and keep a close eye on it. Turn the bread over when the bottom side has browned and broil the other side until golden. Garnish with garlic powder and feta cheese, if desired.

BAZLAMA - TURKISH FLAT BREAD

Preparation: 30 Minutes

Cook: 15 Minutes

Servings: 4

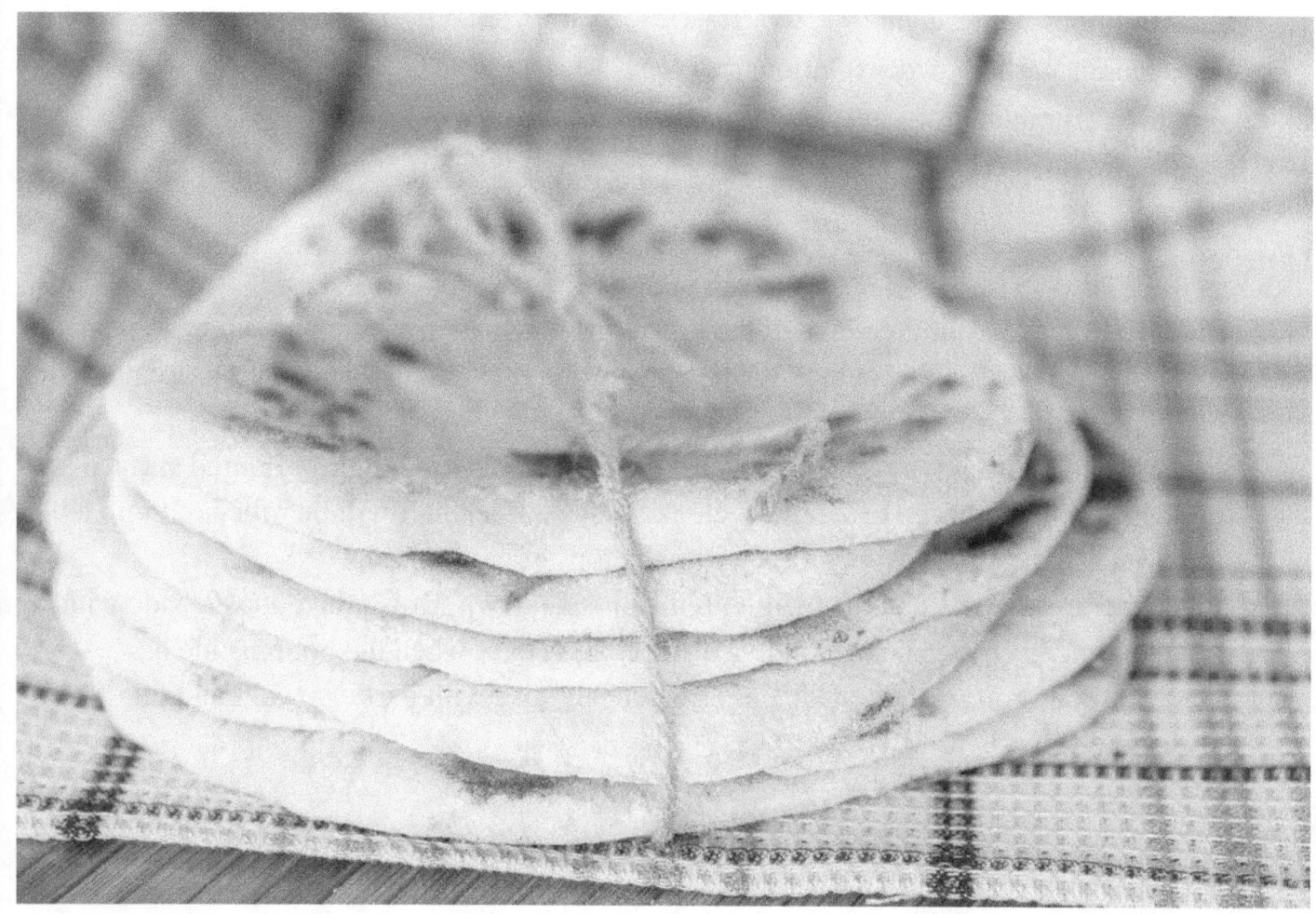

After coming to Turkey, we learned how to make Bazlama, a simple and excellent country bread. Normally, it is prepared in an outdoor oven, but it can also be prepared on a stovetop. It's preferable to eat it when it's still warm.

Nutrition

Calories: 505 | Protein: 15.1g | Fat: 3.8g | Cholesterol: 5.6mg

Sodium: 1766.4mg | Carbohydrates: 100.2g

Ingredients

- 4 cups all-purpose flour
- 1 ½ cups warm water
- 1 package active dry yeast
- ½ cup Greek-style yogurt
- 1 tablespoon white sugar
- 1 tablespoon salt

Instructions

1. In a bowl of warm water, dissolve the yeast, sugar, and salt. In a large mixing bowl, combine the flour, water, and yogurt. Although the dough will be soft, it will not be sticky. Form the dough into a ball and place it on a lightly floured surface. Allow the dough to rise for three hours at room temperature, covered with a wet cloth.
2. Divide the dough into four equal parts. As if you were making pizza dough, form the dough into circles and flatten each one. Allow the dough to rest for fifteen minutes after covering it with a moist cloth.
3. Over medium-high heat, heat a cast-iron skillet or griddle. Place one dough round in the skillet and bake for 1 minute, or until brown spots develop on the bottom. Bake for another minute after flipping the bread. To keep the bread warm, remove it from the oven and wrap it in a clean kitchen towel.
4. Rep with the rest of the dough circles. Any leftover flatbreads must be stored in an airtight container.

PEPPY'S PITA BREAD

Preparation: 30 Minutes

Cook: 15 Minutes

Servings: 8

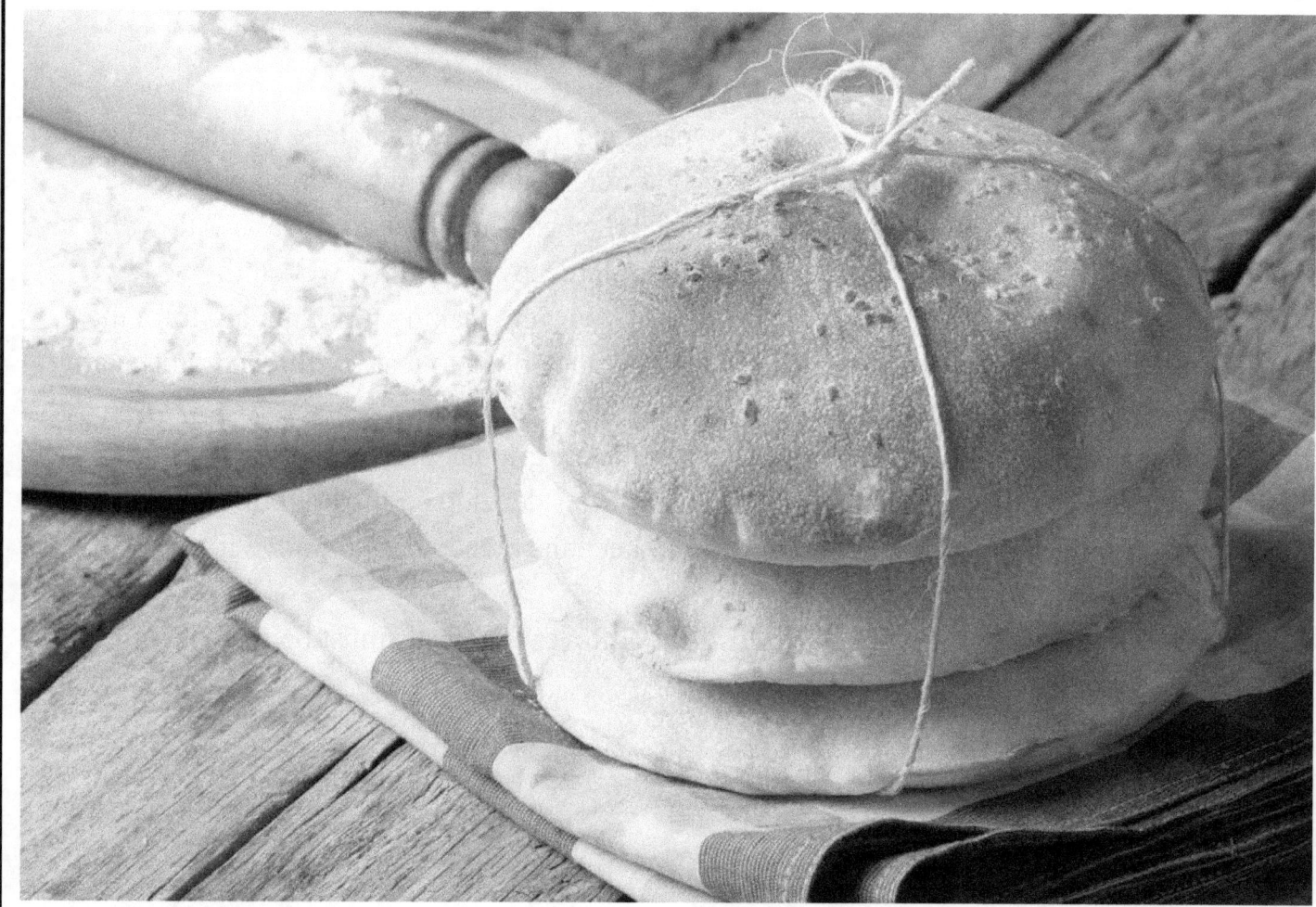

Using this simple method, you can bake fresh pita-style bread in your oven.

Nutrition

Calories: 191 | Protein: 5.1g | Fat: 2.2g | Sodium: 293mg | Carbohydrates: 36.8g

Ingredients

- 1 tablespoon vegetable oil
- 1 ½ teaspoon active dry yeast
- 1 ½ teaspoon white sugar
- 1 ⅛ cups warm water
- 3 cups all-purpose flour
- 1 teaspoon salt

Instructions

1. Place all ingredients in the bread machine's bread pan, select the Dough setting, and start the machine. The machine will sound when the dough has risen sufficiently.
2. On a lightly floured surface, roll out the dough. Roll the dough into a 12-inch rope by gently stretching it. Cut the dough into 8 pieces using a sharp knife. Make a smooth ball out of each. Roll each ball into a 6 to a 7-inch circle using a rolling pin. Place on a lightly floured countertop and set aside. Cover with a cloth to keep the heat in. Allow the pitas to rise for about thirty minutes or until they are somewhat puffy.
3. Preheat the oven to 500 degrees Fahrenheit. On a wire cake rack, arrange 2 or 3 pitas. Place the cake rack on top of the oven rack. Preheat oven to 400°F and bake pitas for four to five minutes, or until puffed and golden brown on top. Remove pitas from the oven and place them in a sealed brown paper bag or a damp kitchen towel until they are tender. After the pitas have softened, cut them in half or split the top edge to make half or full pitas. They can be kept in the refrigerator for several days or frozen for one or two months in a plastic bag.

FOCACCIA ALLA GENOVESE

Preparation: 2 weeks

Cook: 35 Minutes

Servings: 4

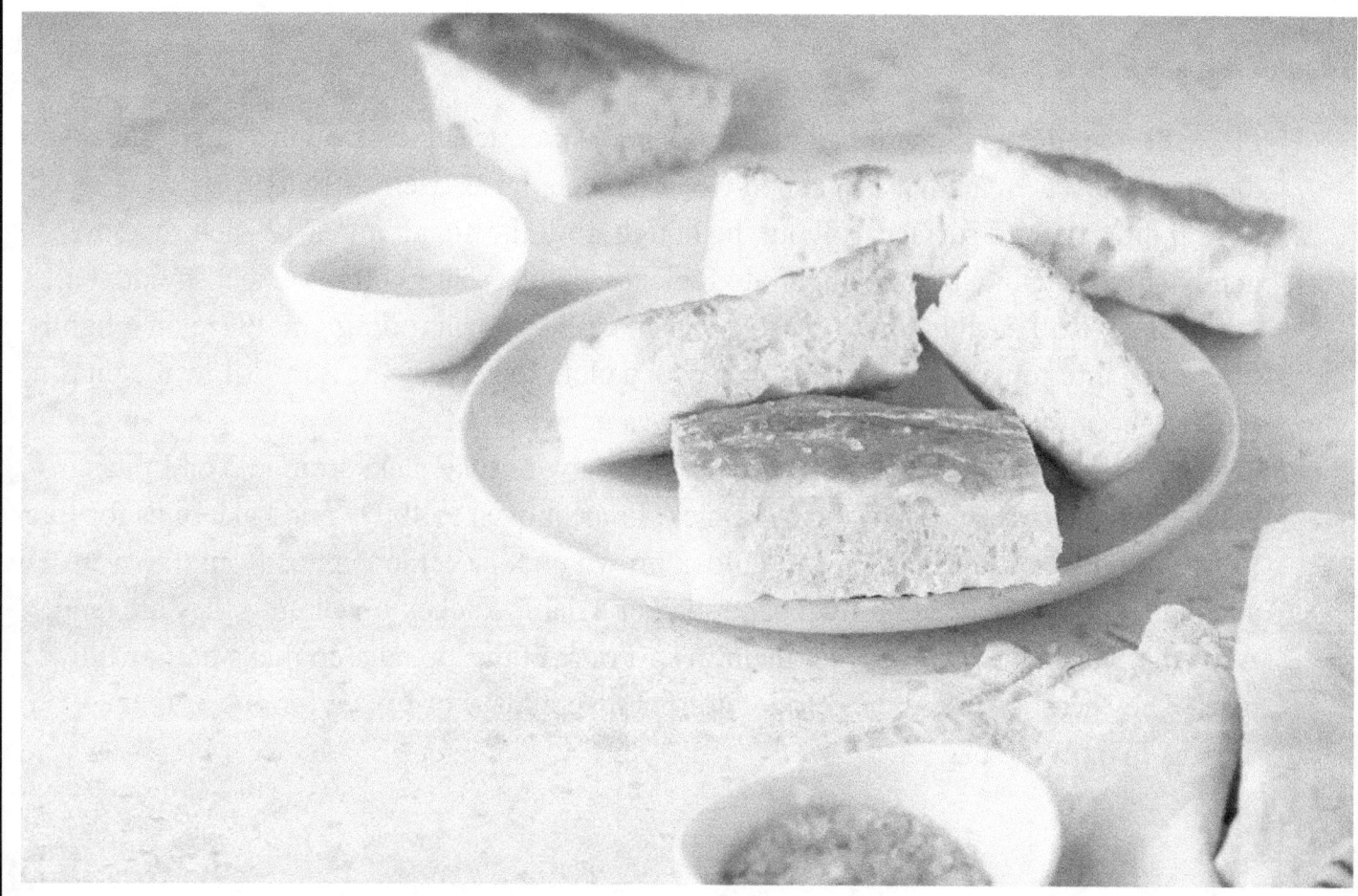

This is a typical Genoese flatbread made with olive oil. It takes a long time to create, but the extra rising period imparts a fantastic taste to the bread.

Nutrition

Calories: 377 | Protein: 10.6g | Fat: 8.2g | Sodium: 294.5mg | Carbohydrates: 63.4g

Ingredients

- ½ cup cold water
- ½ cup warm water
- 2 ½ cups unbleached bread flour
- 1 tablespoon additional extra-virgin olive oil for brushing
- 1 tablespoon extra-virgin olive oil
- 2 teaspoons cornmeal for dusting
- ½ teaspoon active dry yeast
- ½ teaspoon salt
- 1/4 cup biga

Instructions

1. In a small bowl, pour 1/2 cup warm water and sprinkle yeast on top. Allow for ten minutes for the yeast to absorb.
2. In a large mixing bowl, combine flour and salt. Pour the cold water, yeast mixture, 1 tablespoon olive oil, and biga into the well in the center. Using a firm wooden spoon, mix everything together.
3. When the dough has come together, spread it onto a floured surface and knead for twenty minutes. If you want, take a couple of one to two minutes rests. Until the dough is properly kneaded, it will be slightly sticky. Make a ball out of the dough. Place the dough in a clean bowl that has been oiled on the inside. Turn the ball to coat it in oil. Allow it to rise at room temperature until it has doubled in size. This will take about one and a half hours.
4. By folding the edges into the middle and turning the dough over, the top will be smooth once more. Cover the bowl again and let the dough rest for another forty-five minutes, or until it has doubled in size.
5. Turn the dough out onto a floured surface and use your palms to flatten it into an 8-inch square gently. Cover and allow to rise once more.
6. Preheat oven to 425 degrees Fahrenheit. While the oven is heating up, place a baking stone inside. Cornmeal-dusted baker's peel is carefully slid under the dough square. By pressing your fingers about 3/4 of the way into the dough, you may create a dimpled surface. Use water to mist.
7. Sprinkle a little cornmeal on the baking stone's surface. Remove the square from the peel and place it on the baking stone. Spray some water into the hot oven and close the door fast.
8. In a preheated oven, bake for thirty minutes, or until golden brown on top. Remove the pan from the oven and set it to cool on a wire rack. While the Foccacia is still hot, brush the surface with the remaining olive oil.

NONI AFGHANI

Preparation: 15 Minutes

Cook: 25 Minutes

Servings: 8

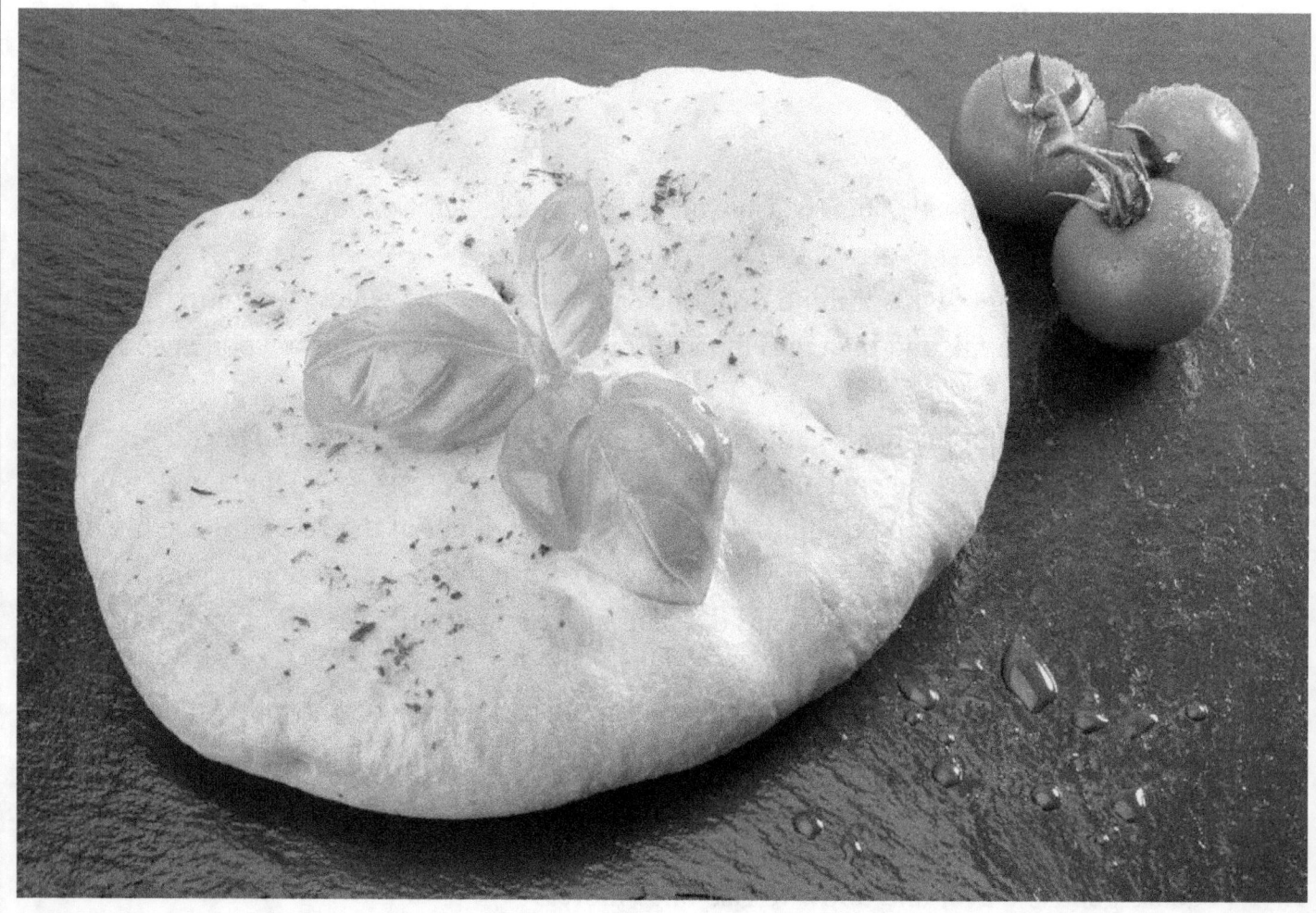

This is a simple flatbread recipe that yields a soft, supple product. This bread, according to my native Afghani acquaintance, tastes better than the traditional bread she buys at the shop. Enjoy!

Nutrition

Calories: 309 | Protein: 7.7g | Cholesterol: 23.3mg | Sodium: 375.3mg

Carbohydrates: 50.1g | Fat: 8.3g

Ingredients

- 1 egg
- ¼ cup corn oil
- 1 tablespoon water
- 1 ½ cups warm water
- 1 ¼ teaspoons salt, or to taste
- 4 cups all-purpose flour
- 1 envelope active dry yeast
- 1 tablespoon white sugar
- 1 tablespoon caraway seed (Optional)

Instructions

1. Combine 1/2 cup warm water and sugar in a small bowl. Sprinkle the yeast on top and set aside for about ten minutes, or until it foams up.
2. In a large mixing bowl, combine flour and salt. In the center of the bowl, make a well and pour in the corn oil and yeast mixture. Continue to add little amounts of water until you have a soft, moist dough that can be handled. Knead the dough for at least five minutes on a floured surface. Return to the bowl, cover with a towel, and let rise for one and half hours or until doubled in size.
3. Preheat the oven to 350°F. Deflate the dough and cut it into eight pieces. Make a ball out of each piece.
4. Roll each ball with a rolling pin on a lightly floured board until it is oval, about 6 inches long, and 1/2 inch thick. Draw three lines on the top of each loaf using a fork or a dull knife. Place the loaves on a baking pan and bake for thirty minutes. Brush the tops of the loaves with the egg mixture and the remaining tablespoon of water. If used, sprinkle caraway seeds on top.
5. In a preheated oven, bake for twenty to twenty-five minutes, or until the loaves are beautiful and golden brown.

LEPINJA (SERBIAN FLATBREAD)

Preparation: 30 Minutes

Cook: 20 Minutes

Servings: 12

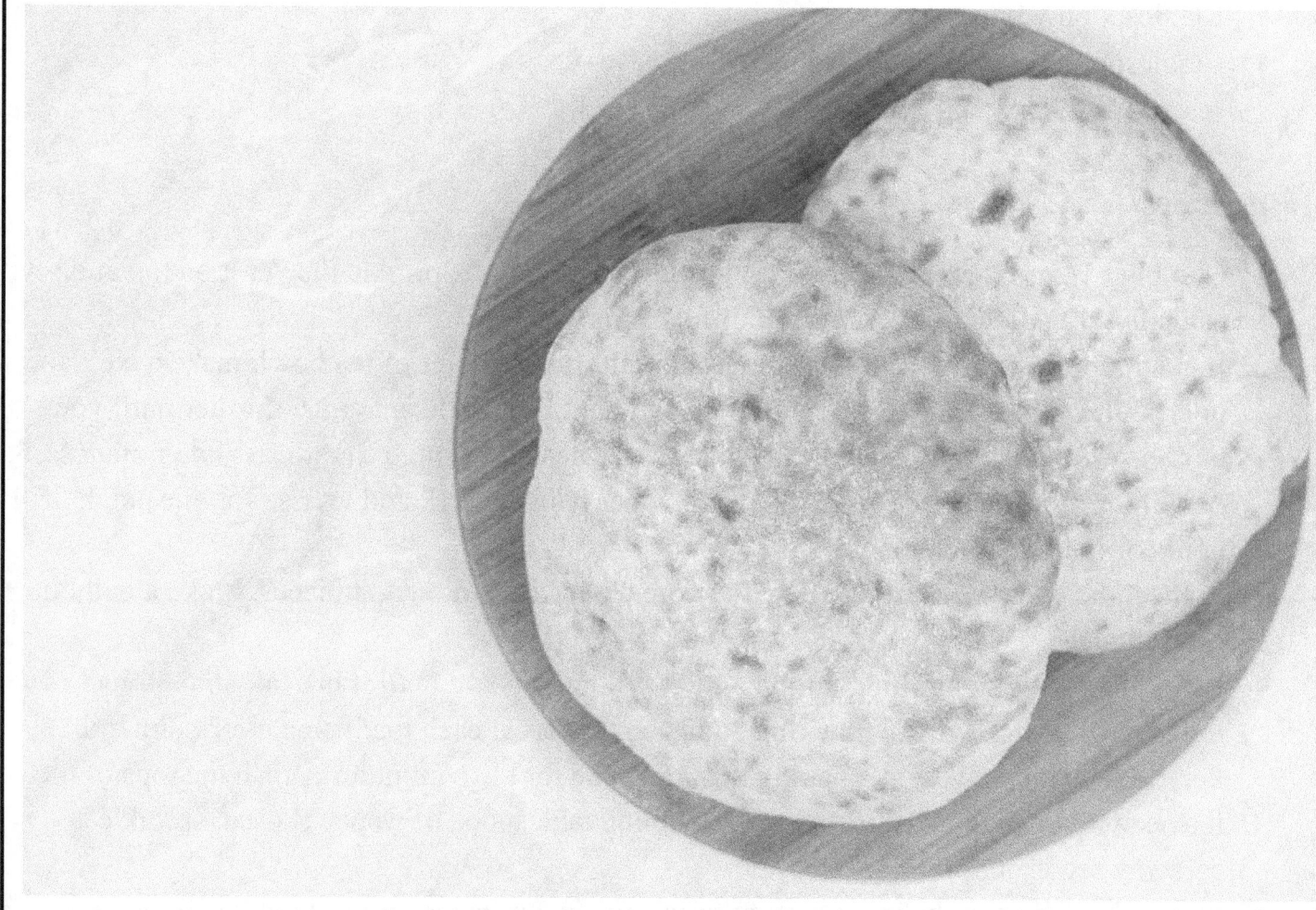

This recipe is unique and easy to prepare instead of others.

Nutrition

Calories: 96 | Protein: 2.8g | Cholesterol: 0.2mg | Sodium: 196.2mg

Carbohydrates: 19.9g | Fat: 0.3g

Ingredients

- 2 ⅓ cups all-purpose flour
- 1 tablespoon white sugar
- 1 cup warm water
- 1 package active dry yeast
- 2 tablespoons warm milk
- 1 teaspoon salt

Instructions

1. In a small bowl, sprinkle the yeast over the warm milk. Allow it to sit for five minutes or until the yeast softens and forms a creamy foam. In a mixing bowl, combine the yeast, warm water, and sugar.
2. In a separate dish, combine the flour and salt; add all but about 1/2 cup of the flour combination to the yeast mixture; mix with your hands until a soft dough forms, gradually adding the remaining flour mixture until it clears the sides of the bowl. Cover the bowl with a light towel and allow the dough to rise until doubled in volume 80 to 95 degrees in a warm location. Deflate the dough by punching it down and turning it out onto a lightly floured work area to knead for about five minutes. Return the dough to the bowl, cover with a light towel, and let it rise for another thirty minutes or until it has doubled in size.
3. Preheat the oven to 400 degrees Fahrenheit. Grease a baking sheet lightly.
4. Deflate the dough and turn it out onto a lightly floured work area to knead lightly. Shape the dough into an oval approximately 1/2-inch thick on the prepared baking sheet. Set aside for about thirty minutes to rise a third time.
5. Cook for twenty to twenty-five minutes in a preheated oven until beautifully browned and hollow when knocked.

NAAN

Preparation: 30 Minutes

Cook: 7 Minutes

Servings: 14

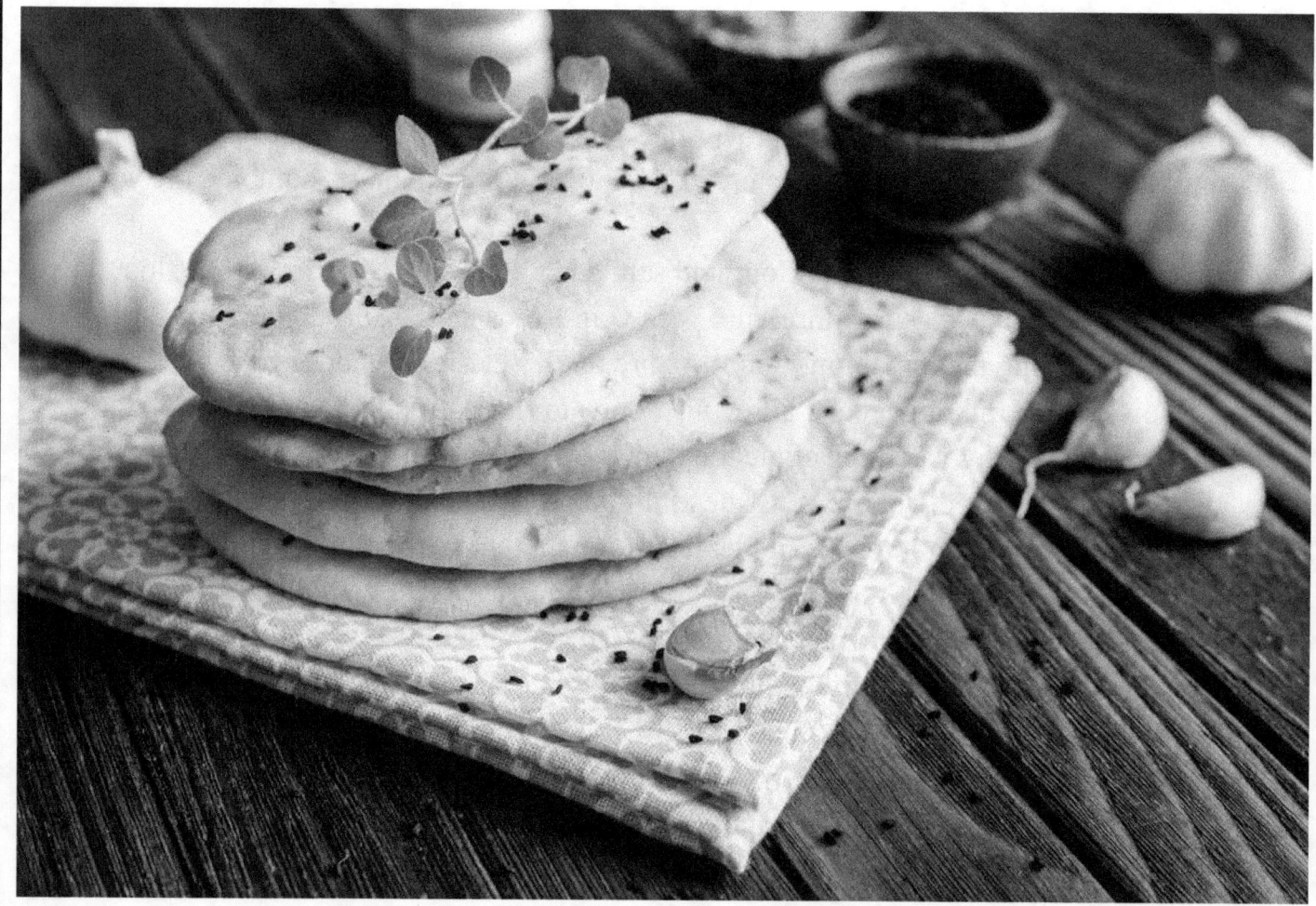

Outside of an Indian restaurant, this recipe makes the greatest naan I've ever had. For my family, we can't get enough of it. They would eat it plain if we didn't serve it with shish kabobs.

Nutrition

Calories: 52 | Protein: 0.8g | Cholesterol: 22.3mg | Sodium 362.7mg

Carbohydrates: 4.1g | Fat: 3.7g

Ingredients

- 4 ½ cups bread flour
- 1 egg, beaten
- ¼ cup white sugar
- 1 package active dry yeast
- 3 tablespoons milk
- 1 cup warm water
- 2 teaspoons salt
- ¼ cup butter, melted
- 2 teaspoons minced garlic (Optional)

Instructions

1. Dissolve yeast in warm water in a large mixing dish. Allow it to sit for ten minutes or until foamy. To produce a soft dough, combine the sugar, milk, egg, salt, and just enough flour. Knead for six to eight minutes, or until smooth, on a lightly floured surface. Set dough aside to rise in a well-oiled basin, covered with a moist cloth. Allow for an hour of rising time or until the dough has doubled in size.
2. Knead in the garlic after punching down the dough. Take little handfuls of dough about the size of a golf ball, and pinch them off. Place on a tray after rolling into balls. Allow thirty minutes for the dough to rise after being covered with a cloth.
3. Preheat the grill to high heat during the second rise.
4. Roll out one dough ball into a thin circle on the grill side. Grill will be lightly oiled. Cook for two to three minutes, or until puffy and gently browned, on the grill. Turnover and brush the uncooked side with butter. Brush the cooked side with butter and cook for another two to four minutes, or until browned. Remove the naan from the grill and repeat the process until all of the naans is cooked.

CHEF JOHN'S PITA BREAD

Preparation: 30 Minutes

Cook: 10 Minutes

Servings: 8

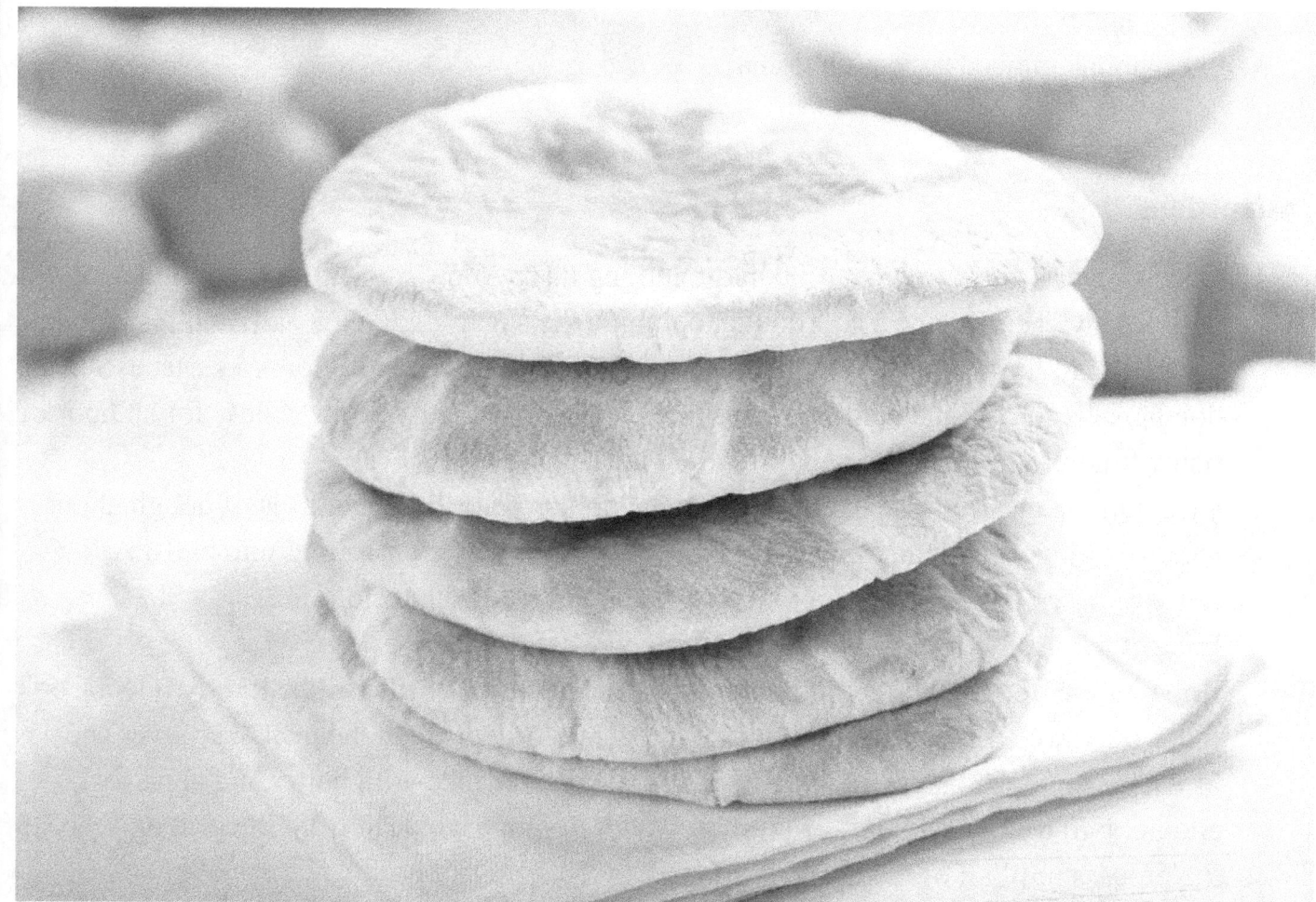

Unlike many other baked goods that are better from a bakery, this is so far better than what you can purchase in the supermarket that it's not even close. It's not only great to eat, but it's also really simple to prepare

Nutrition Facts

Calories: 187 | Fat: 3.6g | Sodium: 510.9mg | Protein: 4.8g | Carbohydrates: 33.1g

Ingredients

- 1 cup all-purpose flour
- 1 ½ tablespoon olive oil
- 1 ¾ cups all-purpose flour, or more as needed
- 1 package active dry yeast
- 1 cup warm water
- 1 teaspoon olive oil, divided
- 1 ¾ teaspoons salt

Instructions

1. In the stand mixer's work bowl, combine yeast, 1 cup warm water, and 1 cup flour. Add all ingredients to a mixing bowl and set aside for fifteen to twenty minutes to allow the dough to rise and form a loose sponge. The mixture will foam and bubble.
2. Pour 1 1/2 tablespoons olive oil and salt into a sponge; add 1 3/4 cup flour. Using a dough hook attachment, mix low speed until dough is soft, pliable, and somewhat sticky. If the dough begins to stick to the sides of the bowl, gradually add up to 1/4 cup extra flour.
3. Knead dough on low speed for five to six minutes, or until somewhat springy and soft. Form a ball out of the dough on a floured work surface.
4. Using 1/4 teaspoon olive oil, wipe the interior of the bowl. Turn dough in a bowl to coat with a thin layer of oil; cover with foil and set aside for two hours, or until the dough has doubled in size.
5. Place the dough on a floured work surface after removing it from the bowl. Lightly pat into a 1-inch thick flat form. Cut the dough into 8 pieces with a knife.
6. Pull dough from the sides and tuck the ends underneath the bottom of each piece to form a little round ball with a smooth top.
7. Allow dough balls to rest for thirty minutes after covering with lightly oiled plastic wrap.
8. Dust a work surface and the top of a dough ball with flour, then gently massage the dough ball flat with your fingertips to form a flat, round bread approximately 1/4 inch thick. Allow five minutes for the dough to rest. Rep with the rest of the dough balls.
9. Place the remaining 3/4 teaspoon olive oil in a cast-iron skillet over medium-high heat. Place pita bread in a heated skillet and cook for three minutes, or until the bread puffs up, and the bottom has brown patches and blisters. Cook for another two minutes on the other side before flipping back to the original side to finish cooking for another thirty seconds. Pita bread will rise and fill with hot air as it cooks.

LONG-FERMENTATION BREAD

Preparation: 50 Minutes

Cook: 1 Hour

Servings: 24

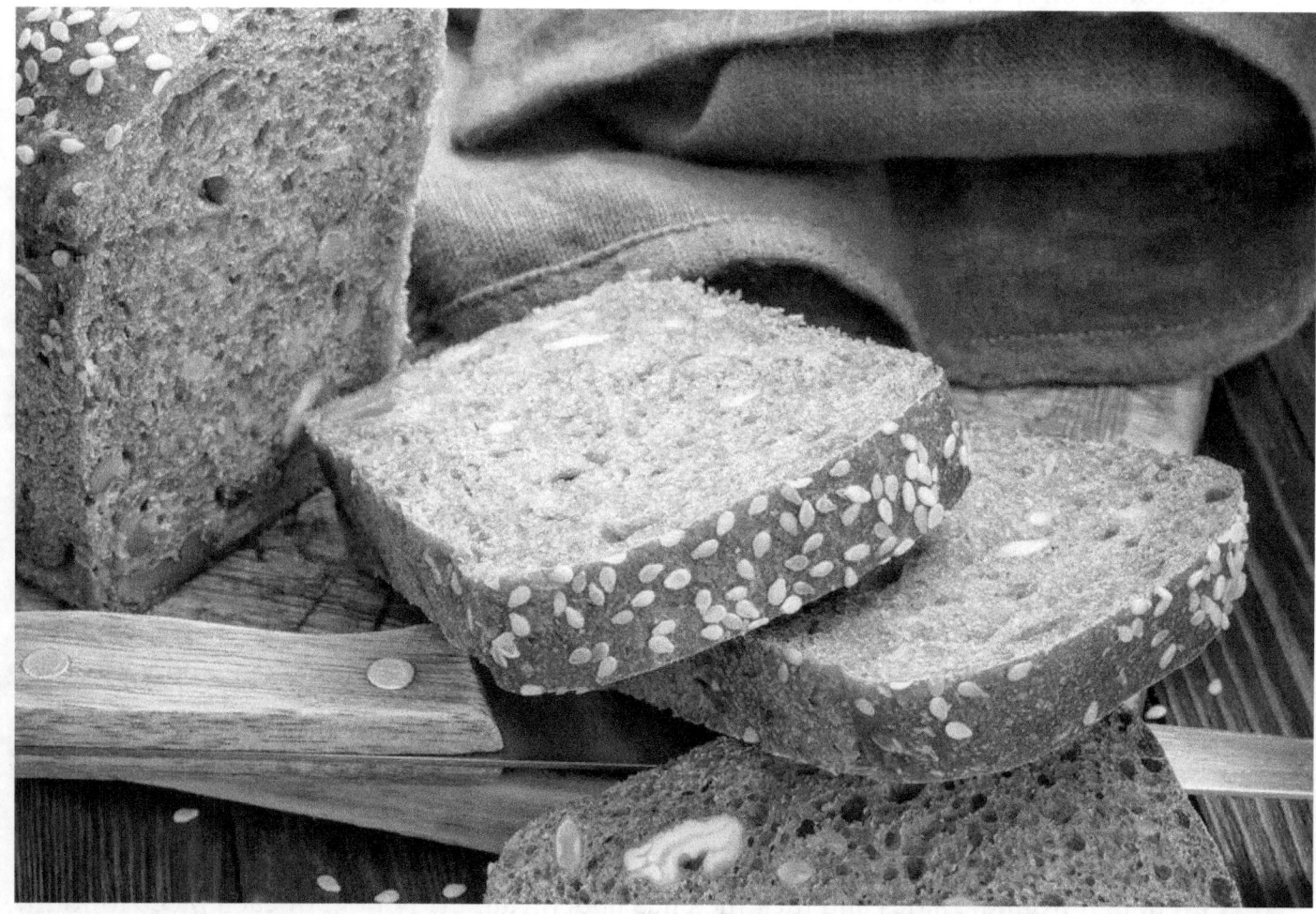

This is a no-knead bread recipe that I created, drawing inspiration from various recipes as well as my own tweaks. The grains soften and swell throughout the long fermentation time, giving the bread a nourishing and gratifying flavor and texture. It features a soft crumb and a chewy crust that crisps up when toasted. This bread is handier because it may be mixed one day ahead of time and cooked the next. The long fermenting process releases the grain's nutrients and improves the bread's flavor.

Nutrition

Calories: 188 | Protein: 6.8g | Fat: 5.1g | Cholesterol: 8.5mg | Sodium: 506.8mg

Carbohydrates: 29.9g

Ingredients

- 5 cups water, 1 egg
- 4 cups whole wheat flour
- 1 tablespoon water, or as needed
- 6 tablespoons vegetable oil
- 6 tablespoons coconut sugar
- 2 tablespoons kosher salt
- 2 cups steel-cut oats
- 5 cups bread flour
- ¾ cup nonfat dry milk powder
- ¾ teaspoon active dry yeast
- 2 tablespoons all-purpose flour, or as needed
- 3 tablespoons raw apple cider vinegar
- 2 tablespoons flax seeds, crushed (optional), 3 tablespoons vital wheat gluten (optional)

Instructions

1. Over medium heat, heat a heavy skillet. Cook, constantly stirring, until the steel-cut oats are lightly toasted, about five minutes. Remove the pan from the heat.
2. In the bowl of a stand mixer fitted with a paddle attachment, combine bread flour, whole wheat flour, toasted steel-cut oats, dry milk, sugar, gluten, salt, flax seeds, and yeast. 5 cups water, 5 cups oil, and 5 cups vinegar mix on low speed until all ingredients have been moistened.
3. In a clean, greased bowl, place the dough. Wrap the dish in plastic wrap. Allow it to rise in a warm location for one to two hours or until doubled in volume.
4. Four–six times, stretch and fold the dough. Return to bowl, cover, and chill for sixteen to eighteen hours.
5. Remove two to four hours before baking from the refrigerator. Sprinkle flour on top of the dough and turn it out onto a well-floured board. Cut the dough in half and flatten each piece. Like an envelope, fold in all four corners and push the edges into the dough. Each piece will be shaped into a loaf with the smooth side facing out. Cover with a non-terry towel and place in two loaf pans. Preheat the oven to 500 degrees Fahrenheit. To make steam for the bread, place a pan of water on the lowest rack.
6. In a small bowl, whisk together the egg and 1 tablespoon of water. Apply the egg wash to the tops of the loaves. Bake for fifteen minutes in a preheated oven until golden brown. Carefully remove the pan of water from the oven and tent the loaves with aluminum foil tents. Continue baking for forty-five to sixty minutes more, or until an instant-read thermometer inserted into a loaf registers 200 to 205 degrees F. Remove the loaves from the pans and set them to cool on a wire rack.

NO-KNEAD WHOLE WHEAT BREAD WITH SORGHUM FLOUR

Preparation: 20 Minutes

Cook: 40 Minutes

Servings: 12

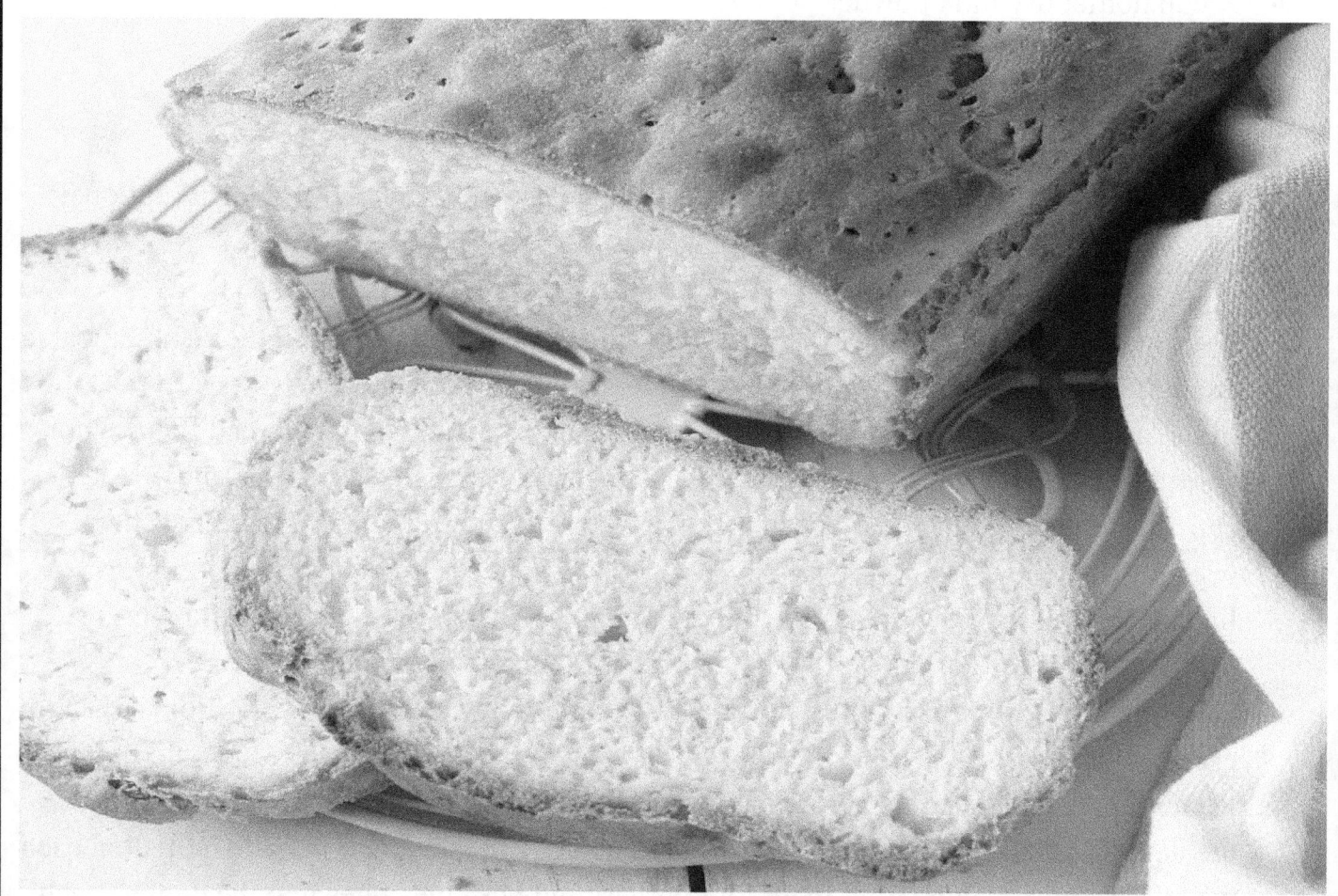

With whole wheat and sorghum flours, this is a delicious no-knead artisan bread alternative. No-knead bread is simple to create, even if you are not a skilled baker. All you need is a Dutch oven.

Nutrition

Calories: 133 | Protein: 5g | Fat: 0.4g | Sodium: 99mg | Carbohydrates: 28g

Ingredients

- 2 cups whole wheat flour
- 1 ½ cups sorghum flour
- ½ package active dry yeast
- 2 tablespoons whole-wheat flour, divided
- 1 ½ cups lukewarm water, or more as needed
- ½ teaspoon salt

Instructions

1. In a small b0wl, dissolve yeast in 1 1/2 cups lukewarm water. Allow five minutes for the mixture to bubble.
2. In a big plastic container with a cover, combine 2 cups whole wheat flour, sorghum flour, and salt. With a wooden spoon, stir in the yeast mixture, adding extra water if the dough is not equally saturated. Allow it to rise in a warm, draft-free environment for about two hours or until doubled in volume.
3. One tablespoon of whole wheat flour is dusted on a cutting board. Turn the dough out onto the board and knead it with your hands for a few minutes. Form the dough into a circular loaf. Place the remaining 1 tablespoon flour in a bowl with a clean dishtowel. Place the dough in the bowl and cover with the dish towel's ends; let rest for one and half hours or until nearly doubled in volume.
4. After the dough has risen for forty-five minutes, preheat the oven to 450 degrees F. After twenty-five minutes, place a covered Dutch oven inside.
5. Using oven mitts, remove the hot Dutch oven from the oven. Using floured hands, carefully place the dough within. Place the hot lid on top.
6. Preheat the oven to 350°F and bake the bread covered for thirty minutes. Remove the lid and bake for another ten minutes, or until the top is golden brown. Using oven mitts, lift the bread out of the Dutch oven and tap the bottom; if it sounds hollow, the bread is done. Allow for at least one hour of cooling time.

ARTISAN NO-KNEAD BREAD WITH AMARANTH

Preparation: 20 Minutes

Cook: 43 Minutes

Servings: 12

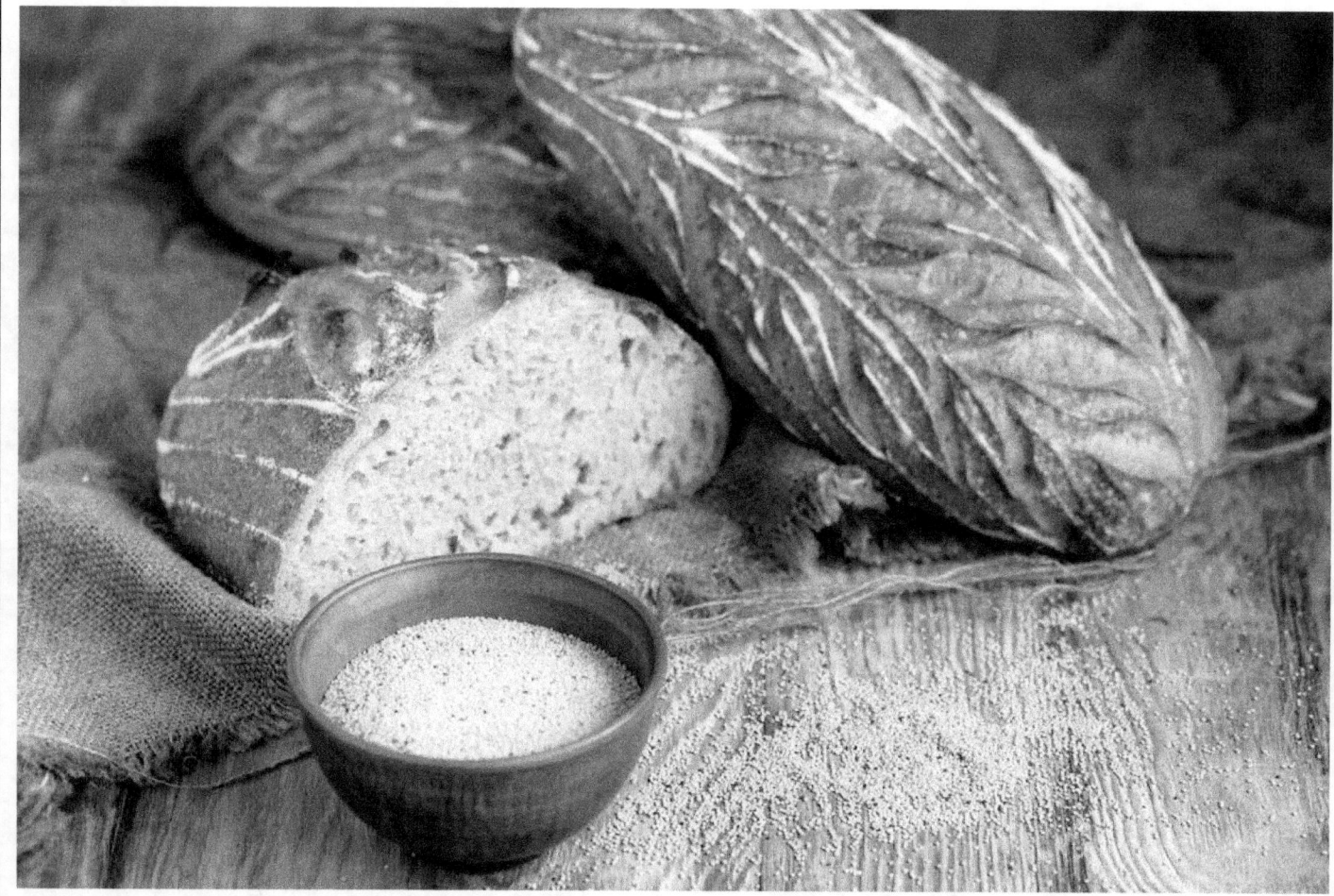

This was my first-time baking using amaranth, and its nutty flavor immediately smote me. This recipe yields one enormous loaf, cut in half and frozen the other half.

Nutrition

Calories: 300 | Protein: 9.9g | Fat: 1.9g | Sodium: 588.5mg | Carbohydrates: 60g

Ingredients

- 2 ¾ cups water
- 4 ½ cups all-purpose flour
- 1 ½ cups bread flour
- 1 tablespoon all-purpose flour
- 1 cup amaranth
- 1 tablespoon salt
- 4 ½ teaspoons active dry yeast

Instructions

1. Heat a skillet over medium heat, add the amaranth; cook and stir for three to five minutes, or until browned and aromatic. Remove from the heat and set aside to cool.
2. In a small dish, dissolve yeast in 1/4 cup lukewarm water. Allow five minutes for the mixture to bubble.
3. In a large plastic container with a cover, stir together the remaining 2 1/2 cups water, toasted amaranth, yeast mixture, all-purpose flour, bread flour, and salt with a wooden spoon until well blended. Cover and let rise in a warm, draft-free place for about two hours or until doubled in volume.
4. 1 tablespoon all-purpose flour, dusted on a cutting board. Turn the dough out onto the board and knead with floured hands for a few minutes. Make a ball out of it.
5. Using parchment paper, line a large mixing basin. Place the dough in the bowl and cover with a clean dish towel; let rise for one and half hours or until nearly doubled in volume.
6. After the dough has risen for forty-five minutes, preheat the oven to 450 degrees F. After twenty-five minutes, place a covered Dutch oven inside.
7. Using oven mitts, remove the hot Dutch oven from the oven. Carefully place the dough inside, raising it with the parchment paper. With kitchen shears, cut any parchment paper that is poking out of the Dutch oven. Place the hot lid on top.
8. Preheat the oven to 350°F and bake the bread covered for thirty minutes. Remove the lid and bake for another 10 minutes, or until the top is golden brown. With oven mitts, lift the bread out of the Dutch oven and tap the bottom; if it sounds hollow, the bread is done. Allow it to cool on a wire rack for at least one hour.

DUTCH OVEN CARAWAY RYE BREAD

Preparation: 15 Minutes

Cook: 35 Minutes

Servings: 12

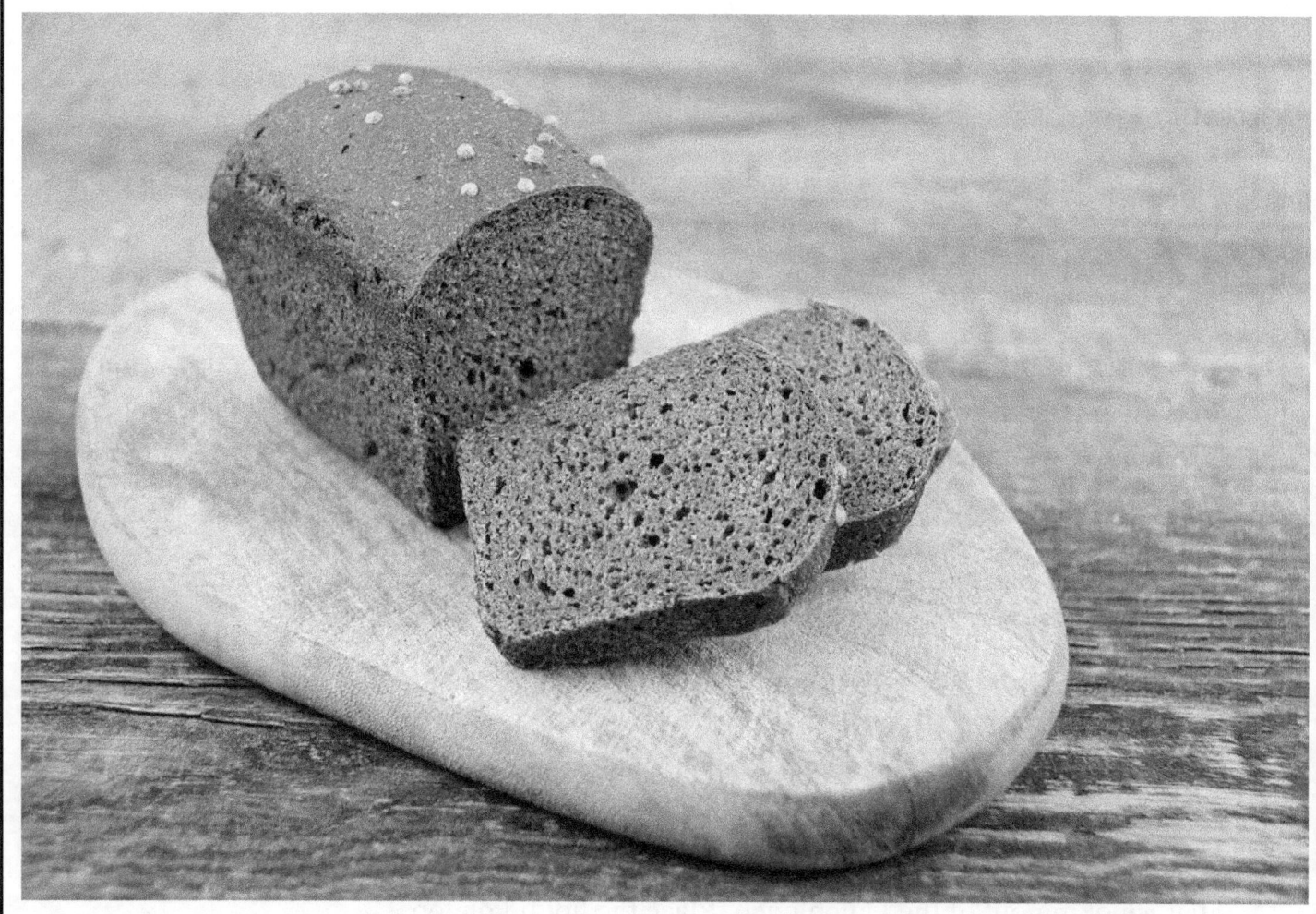

Caraway rye bread made to your specifications! There's no kneading and no double-rise in this no-fail recipe. It's always perfect.

Nutrition

Calories: 145 | Protein: 5g | Cholesterol: 0.2mg | Sodium: 327.6mg

Carbohydrates: 29.6g | Fat: 0.8g

Ingredients

- 1 ¾ cups warm water
- 2 cups light rye flour
- 2 teaspoons white sugar
- 2 cups bread flour
- 2 tablespoons caraway seeds
- 2 teaspoons flaked kosher salt, crushed
- ⅜ teaspoon active dry yeast
- ¼ cup buttermilk
- 1 ½ tablespoon vital wheat gluten (optional)

Instructions

1. In a large bowl, combine rye flour, bread flour, buttermilk, caraway seeds, vital wheat gluten, and kosher salt.
2. In a mixing bowl, whisk together the water, sugar, and yeast until the yeast softens and forms a creamy foam, about five minutes. Stir the yeast mixture into the flour mixture until it is thoroughly combined, and the caraway seeds are spread evenly. Wrap plastic wrap around the bowl and set aside for eighteen hours. Place the dough on a floured work surface. Because it will be somewhat extended, fold the right and left sides into the center. Cover with plastic wrap for Fifteen minutes after turning dough over and carefully tucking corners under a spatula. Remove the plastic wrap, flour the dough, and make small slits on the top to allow the dough to bloom fully.
3. Preheat the oven to 500 degrees Fahrenheit and place a Dutch oven inside.
4. Place dough in a Dutch oven with care, cover immediately, reduce oven temperature to 460 degrees F and bake for thirty to thirty-five minutes, or until bread is cooked through. Transfer the bread from the Dutch oven to the oven rack and bake for an additional five minutes.

RUSTIC BREAD

Preparation: 15 Minutes

Cook: 20 Minutes

Servings: 20

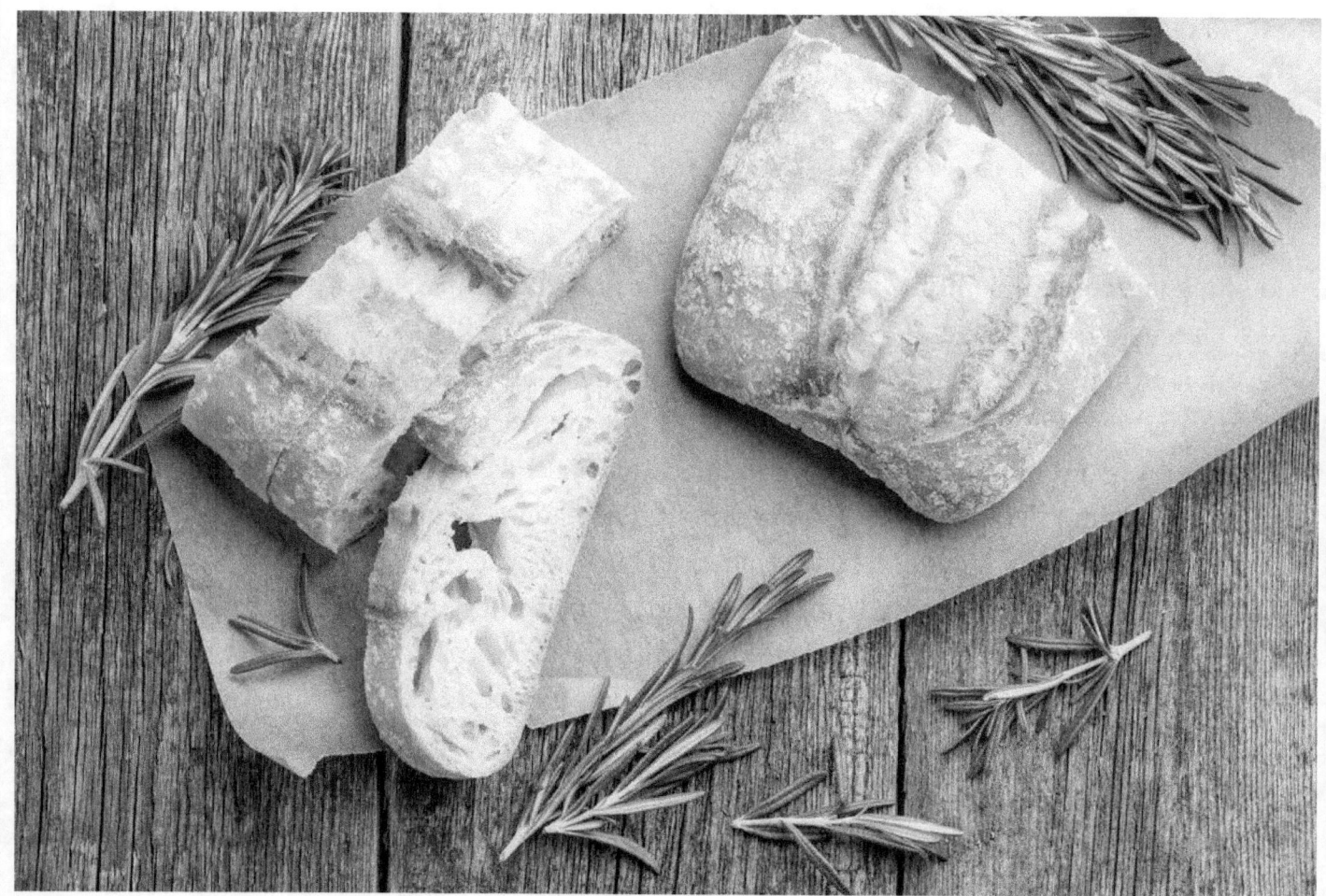

This is the simplest rustic bread recipe I've ever seen. Fortunately, it's also the most delectable. If you only want one loaf, you can make half the recipe, but be warned: it's so addicting that you'll wish you'd made both.

Nutrition

Calories: 162 | Protein: 4.8g | Fat: 0.5g | Sodium: 526.6mg | Carbohydrates 33.7g

Ingredients

- 6 ½ cups all-purpose flour
- ½ cup cornmeal
- 1 ½ tablespoon coarse salt
- 3 cups warm water
- 1 ½ tablespoon active dry yeast

Instructions

1. In a large mixing bowl, whisk together the water, yeast, and salt until the dough gets frothy, about ten minutes. Mix the flour into the yeast mixture until it is completely integrated. The dough will be loose and moist in appearance. Allow sitting for around five hours, loosely covered with a moist towel.
2. Using damp hands, form the dough into two loaves. Place the loaves on a cornmeal-dusted work surface and use a sharp knife to score the tops a few times. Allow thirty to sixty minutes for the loaves to double in size.
3. Preheat the oven to 425 degrees Fahrenheit. Place the loaves on a baking sheet and bake them.
4. Bake for around twenty minutes in a preheated oven, spraying the dough's surface with water now and then.

ENGLISH MUFFIN LOAVES

Preparation: 15 Minutes

Cook: 20 Minutes

Servings: 24

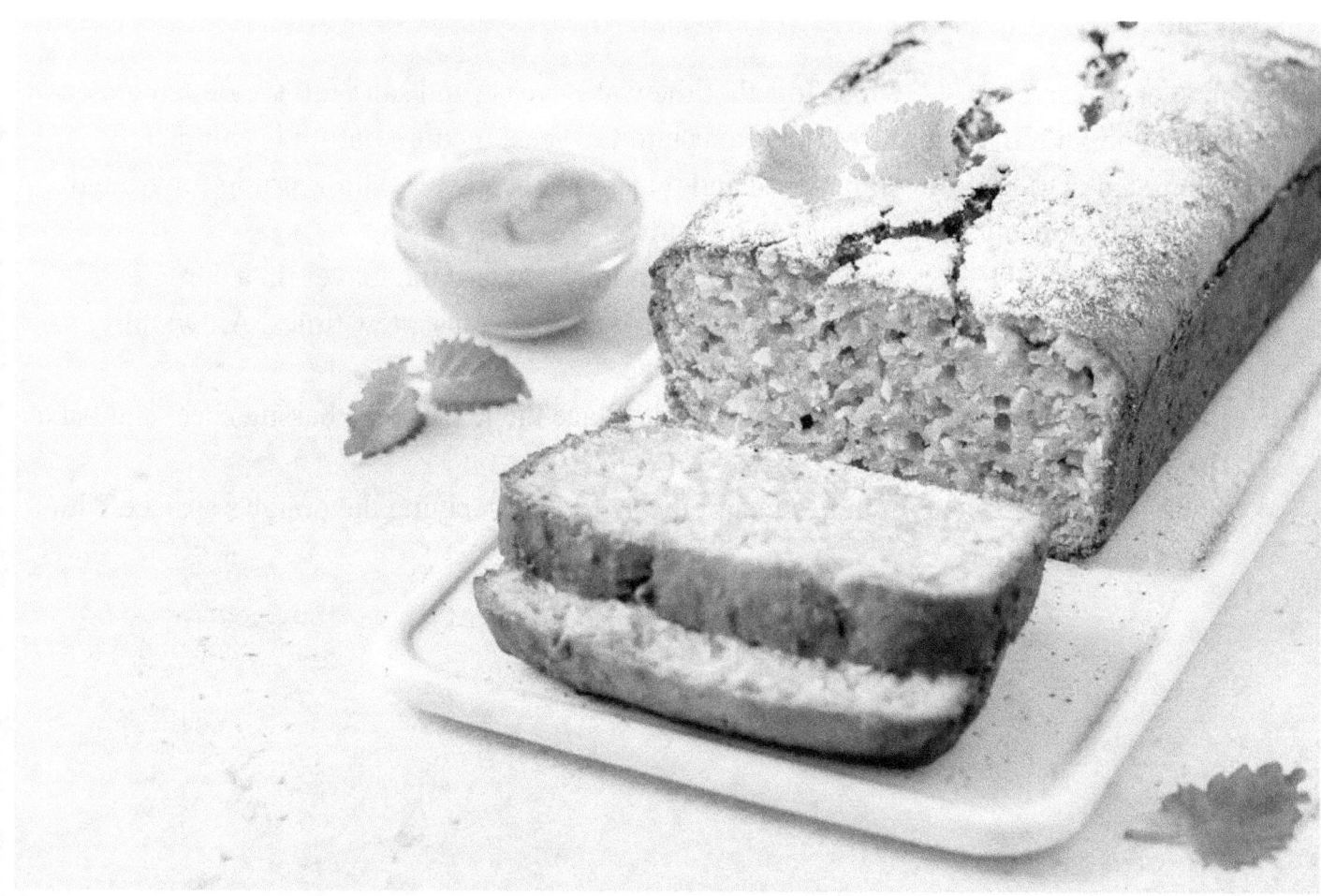

This is a simple yeast bread that requires no kneading. The texture is similar to that of English muffins, making it ideal for toasting.

Nutrition

Calories: 130 | Protein: 4.2g | Fat: 0.7g | Cholesterol: 1.6mg | Sodium: 119.3mg

Carbohydrates: 26.1g

Ingredients

- 2 cups milk
- 6 cups all-purpose flour
- ½ cup water
- 2 packages of active dry yeast
- 1 tablespoon white sugar
- 1 teaspoon salt
- ¼ teaspoon baking soda
- 2 tablespoons cornmeal

Instructions

1. Heat the milk and water in a small pot until very heated.
2. In a large mixing bowl, combine 3 cups flour, yeast, sugar, salt, and soda. Mix in the heated milk and water thoroughly. To produce a stiff batter, stir in enough of the remaining flour. Fill two greased and cornmeal-dusted 9 x 5-inch loaf pans halfway with batter. Cover and set aside for forty-five minutes to rise in a warm location.
3. Preheat the oven to 400 degrees F and bake for twenty-five minutes. Remove from pans as soon as possible and set aside to cool.

GLUTEN-FREE SOURDOUGH RAISIN BREAD

Preparation: 15 Minutes

Cook: 40 Minutes

Servings: 10

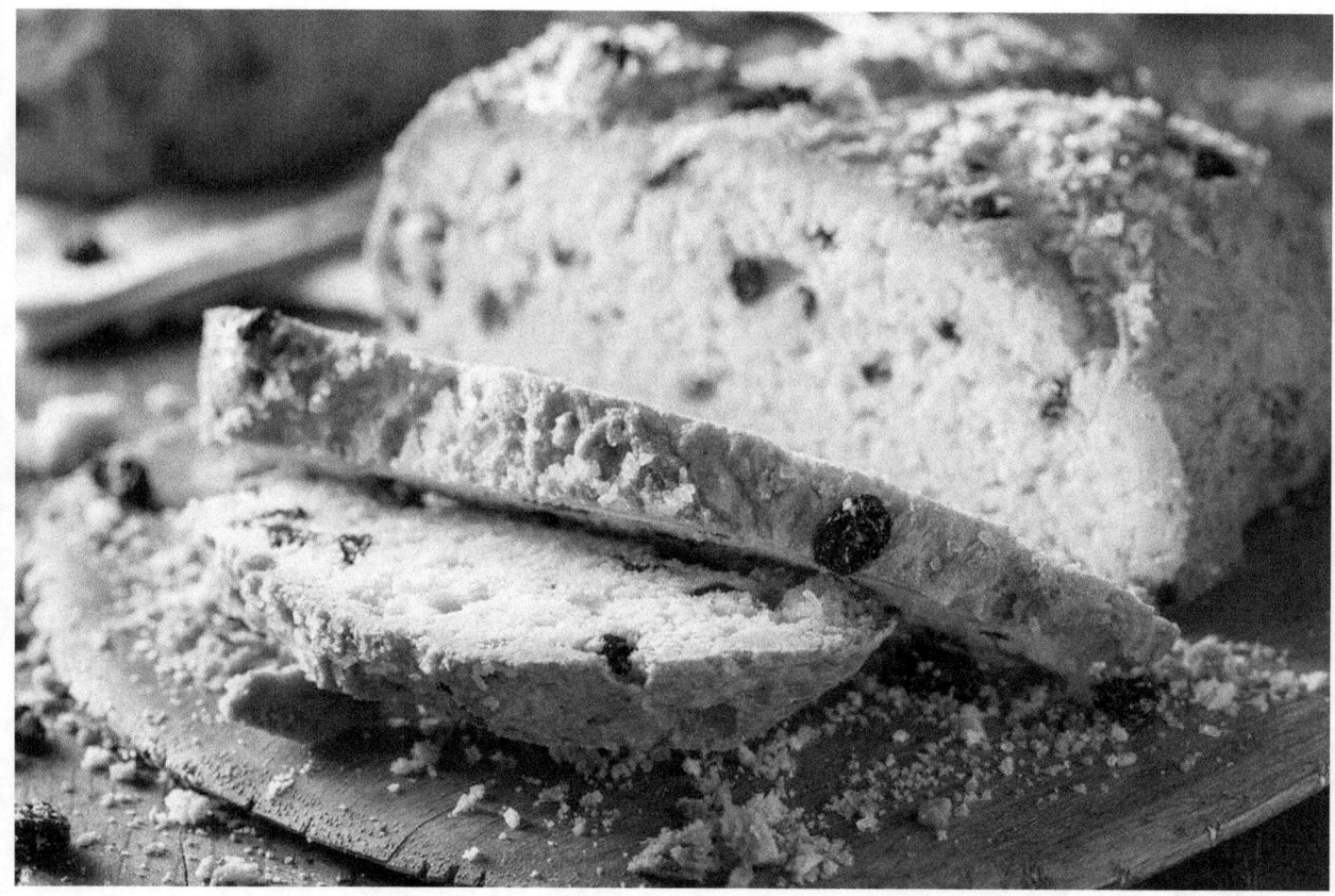

Instead of commercial yeast, use gluten-free sourdough starter trash to make cinnamon raisin bread. During the Covid-19 lockdown, when yeast had vanished from supermarkets, we created this recipe. Because there is no kneading involved, this light and fluffy loaf comes together quickly; it's more like a batter than a dough. Toasted, this bread is wonderful

Nutrition

Calories: 219 | Protein: 6.2g | Fat: 2.9g | Cholesterol: 57.7mg | Sodium: 223.7mg

Carbohydrates: 44.1g

Ingredients

- ¾ cup raisins
- 1 tablespoon ground cinnamon
- ¾ cup whole milk, at room temperature
- ½ cup gluten-free sourdough starter
- 1 teaspoon agave nectar
- 1 teaspoon vanilla extract
- ½ cup buckwheat flour
- 1 pinch cream of tartar
- 3 eggs, lightly beaten
- ¼ cup coconut sugar
- 2 cups gluten-free bread flour mix
- 1 pinch baking soda

Instructions

1. Fill a bowl halfway with lukewarm water and add the raisins. Allow soaking for a while.
2. Using parchment paper, line a loaf pan. In a mixing bowl, combine gluten-free bread flour, buckwheat flour, coconut sugar, cinnamon, cream of tartar, and baking soda.
3. In the bowl of a stand mixer, combine the milk, sourdough starter, and agave nectar. Begin mixing on low and gradually add the flour mixture, 1 tablespoon at a time, until thoroughly incorporated. Mix in the eggs and vanilla extract until thoroughly combined. Drain raisins and fold into the batter
4. Pour the batter into the loaf pan that has been prepared. Using a damp rubber scraper, smooth down the top. Cover the pan loosely with plastic wrap and let rise for about 2 hours, or until about doubled in size. Wrap foil around the dish.
5. Preheat oven to 350 degrees Fahrenheit. Preheat the oven to 350°F and bake the bread for thirty minutes. Remove the foil and bake for another ten minutes or until the bread has browned and reached an internal temperature of 200 degrees. Allow it cool for five minutes in the pan. Remove the bread from the pan and place it on a wire rack to cool completely before slicing.

NO-KNEAD SKILLET OLIVE BREAD

Preparation: 15 Minutes

Cook: 30 Minutes

Servings: 10

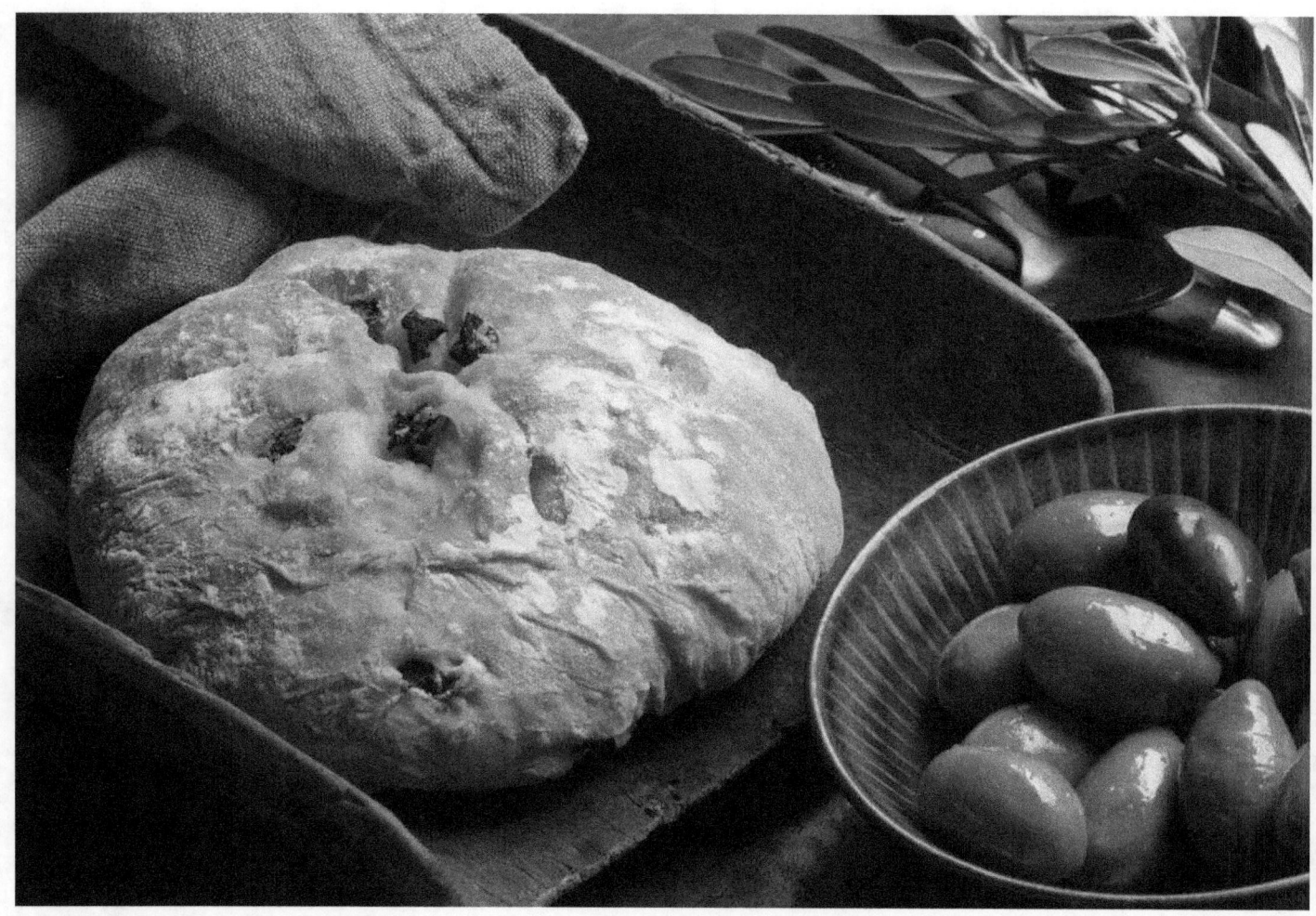

No-knead skillet olive bread is a no-knead, crusty, and tasty no-knead bread filled with marinated olives and garlic.

Nutrition

Calories: 239 | Protein: 5.9g | Fat: 4.8g | Sodium: 774mg | Carbohydrates: 41.8g

Ingredients

- 1 cup marinated olives - drained, chopped, and herbs and garlic reserved
- 4 ⅓ cups all-purpose flour, divided
- 1 teaspoon garlic powder
- 2 tablespoons olive oil, divided
- 1 teaspoon dried parsley, or as needed
- 2 cups lukewarm water
- 1 package active dry yeast
- ½ tablespoon salt
- coarse salt

Instructions

1. In a large mixing bowl, combine the water and yeast. Add 1 cup flour and 1/2 teaspoon salt in a mixing bowl. Using a wooden spoon, stir until everything is well blended. Combine the olives, saved herbs and garlic, and garlic powder in a mixing bowl. 1 cup at a time, whisk in the remaining flour until fully incorporated. Cover bowl with plastic wrap and place in a warm place for one hour to rise.
2. In an 8-inch cast-iron skillet, pour 1 tablespoon of oil and distribute it around to coat the bottom and sides. Using flour, coat your hands. Remove the plastic wrap from the dough and place it in the preheated skillet, shaping it into a disc. Allow thirty minutes to stand after covering with a kitchen towel.
3. Preheat oven to 400 degrees Fahrenheit
4. Drizzle the remaining oil over the bread, then season with salt and parsley. With a knife, score the top of the bread.
5. Bake in the preheated oven until the top is nicely browned, thirty to thirty-five minutes.
6. Remove the bread from the oven and place it on a wire rack to cool for about twenty minutes before serving.

SLOW COOKER BREAD

Preparation: 15 Minutes

Cook: 2 Hours

Servings: 10

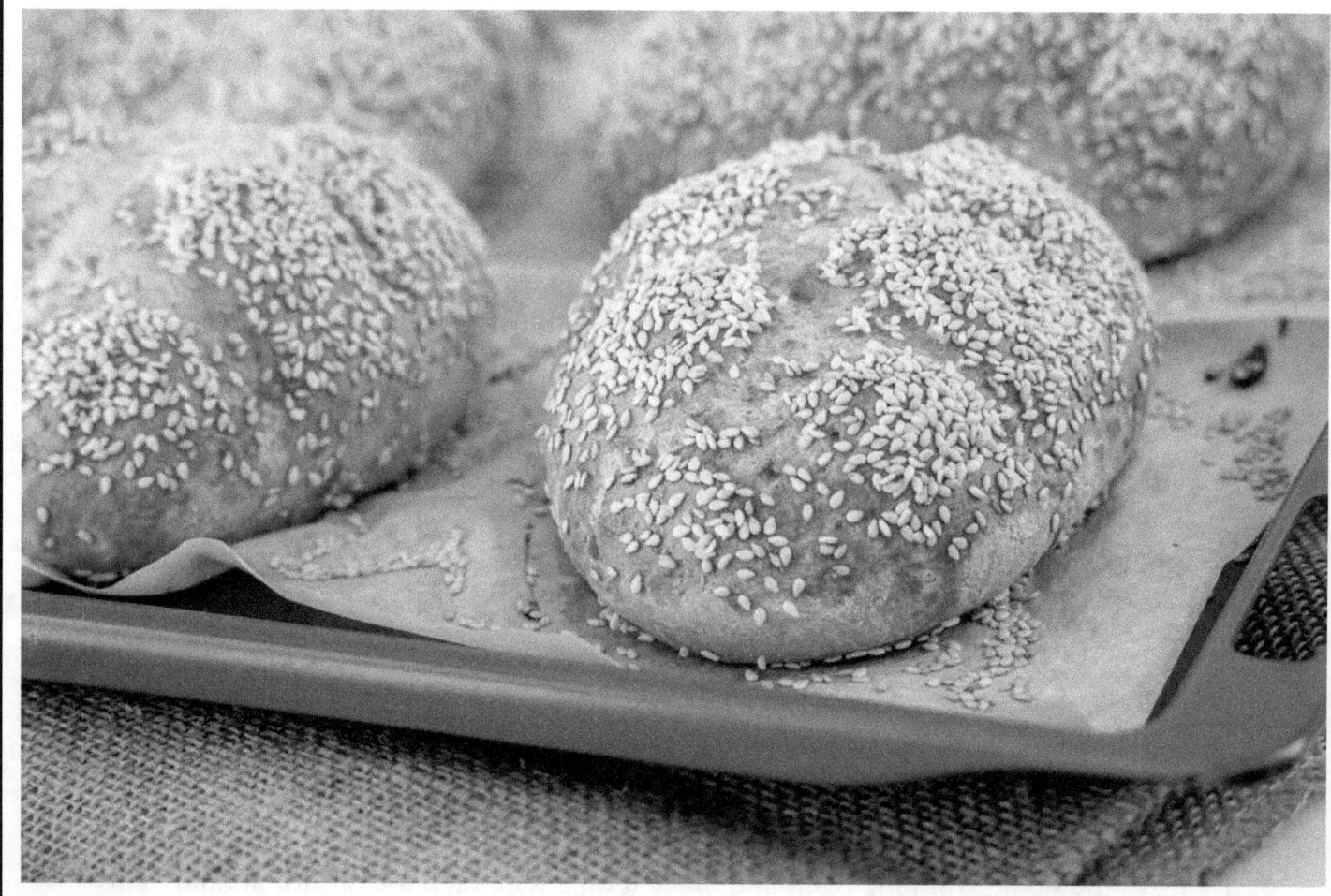

Because this is a no-knead method, the bread made in the slow cooker really turns out to be a decent loaf. It's also rapid because only one rise is required; the second rise takes place in the slow cooker. The addition of seeds or rolled oats enhances the flavor of the bread while also making it easier to remove it from the slow cooker.

Nutrition

Calories: 131 | Protein: 4.5g | Fat: 2.3g | Sodium: 350.9mg | Carbohydrates: 22.8g

Ingredients

- 2 ½ cups bread flour
- 1 ½ teaspoons salt
- 1 cup lukewarm water
- 1 ½ teaspoon active dry yeast
- 1 tablespoon lukewarm water, or more as needed
- ¼ cup sesame seeds
- parchment paper

Instructions

1. In a small dish, combine 1 cup water and yeast and stir until yeast is completely dissolved. Allow ten minutes for the mixture to get frothy or foamy.
2. In a plastic jar with a tight-fitting lid, combine flour and salt. Stir in the yeast mixture with a wooden spoon until it is completely blended and no traces of flour remain. Stir in 1 to 2 tablespoons of water until the dough is tacky but not moist. Place the lid on the container. Allow 1 hour for the dough to rise at room temperature.
3. Set the slow cooker's temperature high. To line the bottom of your slow cooker cut a piece of parchment paper.
4. Using flour, dust a clean work surface. To remove any air pockets, knead the dough slightly with floured hands. Depending on the shape of your slow cooker, shape either a round or oval loaf.
5. On the bottom of the slow cooker, sprinkle some sesame seeds. The remaining seeds will be liberally sprinkled all over the loaf. Cover the dough in the slow cooker with the lid.
6. Cook for two hours on high. During cooking, lift the lid several times to let the steam out. A deep-in-the-loaf instant-read thermometer should read between 200 to 210 degrees F. The bread should be dry and no longer spongy on the surface. Take the loaf out of the oven and tap it on the bottom; it should sound hollow.

NO-KNEAD COUNTRY BREAD

Preparation: 20 Minutes

Cook: 30 Minutes

Servings: 12

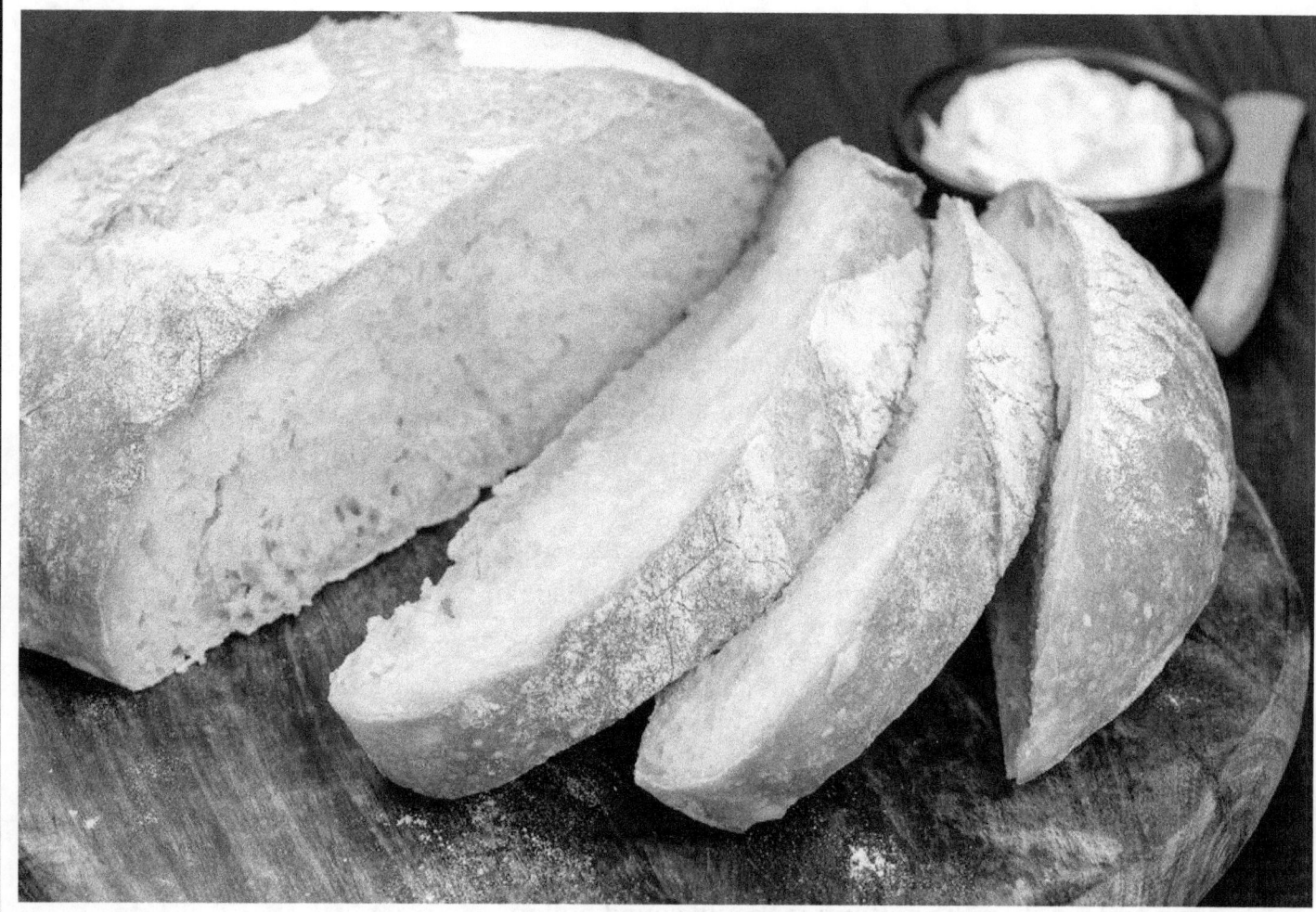

This delectable and beautiful loaf is half recipe, part science experiment, and fun family project for when you're trapped at home with nothing to do. The texture you obtain is wonderful, even though it takes a long time. If preferred, top with butter and jam.

Nutrition

Calories: 143 | Protein: 4.9g | Fat: 0.8g | Sodium: 241.9mg | Carbohydrates: 28.9g

Ingredients

- 2 cups cold water
- ¼ teaspoon active dry yeast
- ½ cup sprouted spelt flour
- 1 ½ teaspoon fine kosher salt
- 3 ½ cups white bread flour

Instructions

1. In a large mixing dish, combine together white bread flour, whole wheat bread flour, and yeast with a wooden spoon. Pour in cold water and stir with a wooden spoon or spatula for three minutes, or until a very moist, sticky dough forms.
2. Mix for another two to three minutes after adding the salt. Scrape the bowl's sides clean. Wrap foil around the dish. Allow dough to rise for eighteen hours at room temperature.
3. With a spatula, deflate the frothy dough by scraping down the sides of the basin and folding the dough over itself twelve times or so, turning the bowl as you go around in a circular motion. With a spatula, scrape the dough onto a very well-floured board. Dust the dough's surface liberally with flour. Flour your hands well, then roll and fold the dough on the table for one to two minutes, or until you've produced a round or oval loaf shape with a smooth surface. Because the dough is quite sticky, you may need to add more flour. The shape isn't as important as the smoothness of the surface. Allow it to rise, uncovered, for two hours or until doubled in size on a Silpat-lined baking sheet. It's usual for the dough to spread out rather than rising. Preheat oven to 450 degrees Fahrenheit.
4. With a very sharp knife or razor, make 1 shallow gash along the middle of the dough, being careful not to deflate the dough too much; the slash is optional. To assist the crust form, lightly spray the surface of the bread with plain water.
5. Bake for thirty minutes in the center of a preheated oven until well browned. Allow it to cool completely before cutting.

BETTER-THAN-BAKERY NO-KNEAD SOURDOUGH

Preparation: 10 Minutes

Cook: 45 Minutes

Servings: 12

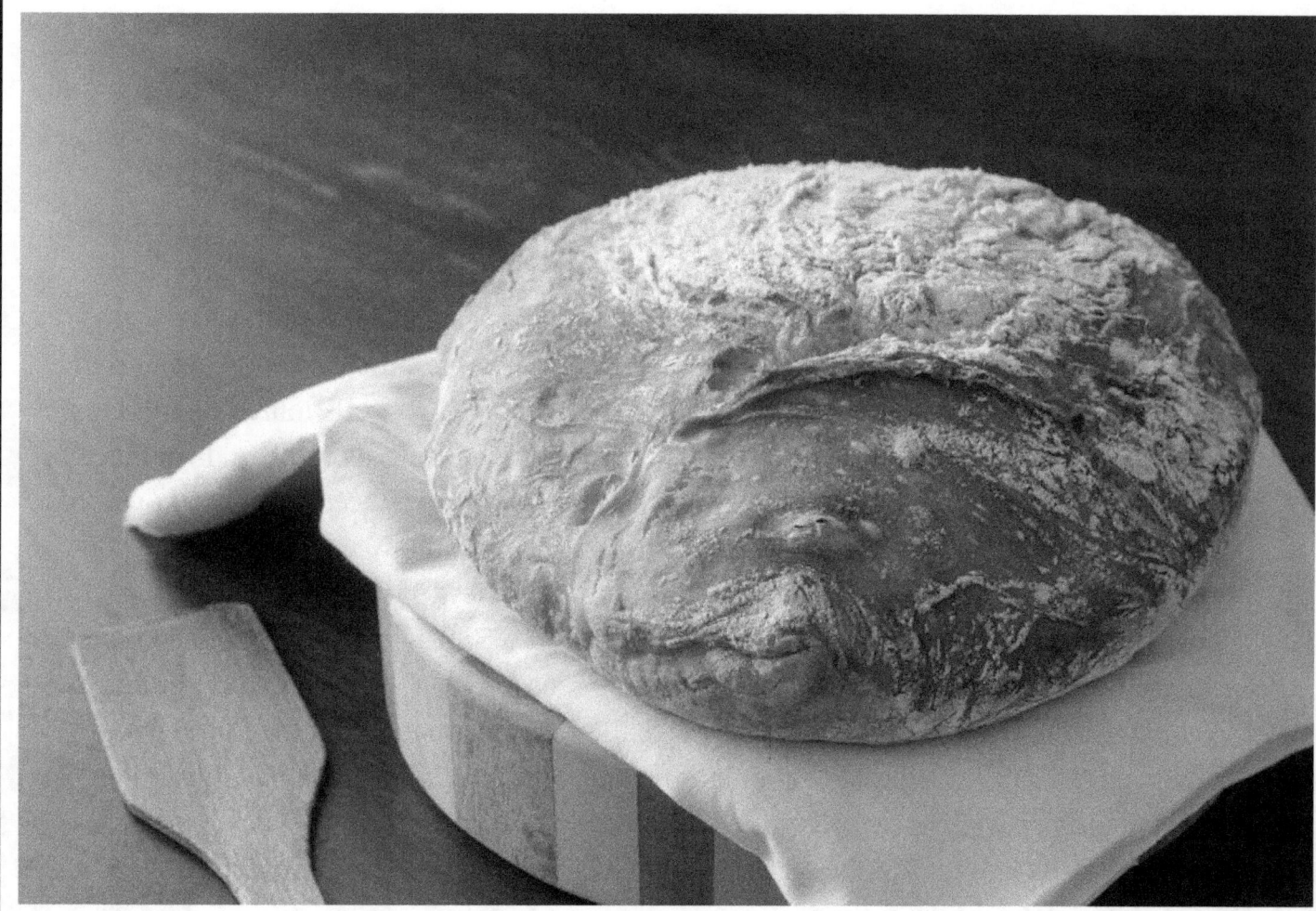

This bread is unbelievably crusty, chewy, and acidic. You'll be surprised at how easy it is to make a professional-looking loaf at home. The crust is glossy and crispy. Crumb is resilient and airy. The baking results in a Dutch oven (placed in your household oven) are very similar to those of a professional bread oven.

Nutrition

Calories: 33 | Protein: 1.4g | Cholesterol: 0.1mg | Sodium: 491.1mg

Carbohydrates: 6.4g | Fat: 0.1g

Ingredients

- 6 cups bread flour
- 1 cup sourdough starter
- 2 ½ teaspoons salt
- 3 cups room-temperature water
- 1 tablespoon cornmeal, or more as needed

Instructions

1. In a large mixing dish, combine the water and salt. Stir in 3 cups bread flour until smooth, then add sourdough starter and whisk rapidly to blend and aerate. Stir in the remaining 3 cups of bread flour until the dough comes together completely.
2. Cover bowl and set aside for twelve to fifteen hours, or until dough is bubbly and risen in volume.
3. Using floured hands, transfer the dough to a well-floured work surface. To coat the dough with flour, turn it many times. Return the dough to an oiled basin and rest for two to three hours, or until it has doubled in size but not collapsed.
4. Preheat an oven-safe, covered Dutch oven for thirty minutes at 450 degrees F.
5. Using oven mitts, carefully remove the Dutch oven and sprinkle cornmeal into the bottom to prevent the dough from sticking.
6. Replace the lid on the Dutch oven and gently roll out the dough from the oiled bowl.

CHEF JOHN'S WHOLE WHEAT CIABATTA

Preparation: 45 Minutes

Cook: 30 Minutes

Servings: 12

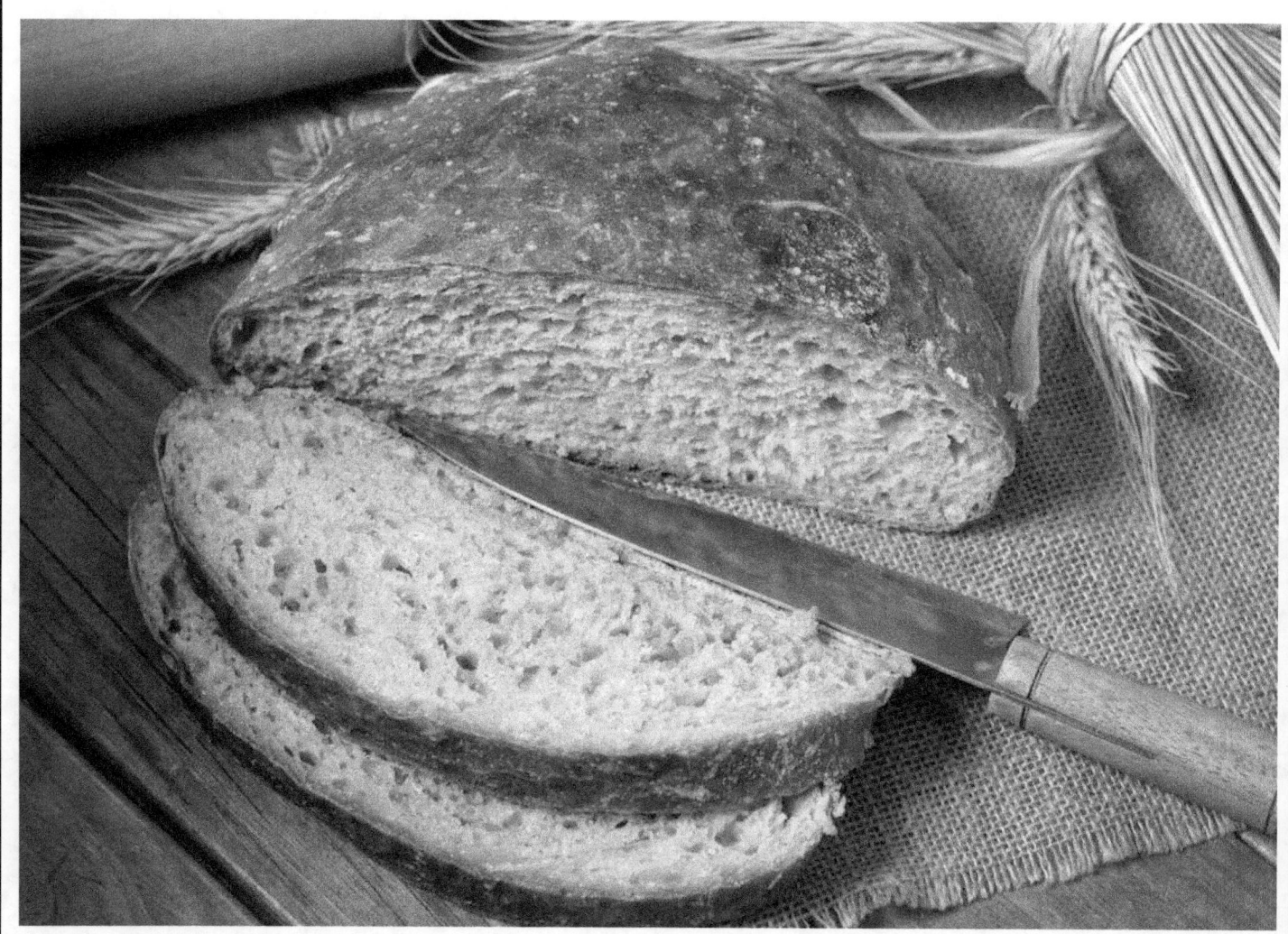

In this recipe, the taste and texture were excellent, and using 50/50 all-purpose flour offered just crusty enough, chewy 'regular' bread texture

Nutrition

Calories: 135 | Protein: 4.5g | Cholesterol: 0.1mg | Sodium: 349.2mg

Carbohydrates: 26.6g | Fat: 1.6g

Ingredients

- 1 cup all-purpose flour
- 1 cup whole wheat flour
- 1 cup warm water
- ½ cup all-purpose flour
- ¼ cup rye flour
- water as needed
- ¼ teaspoon active dry yeast
- ½ cup water at room temperature
- 2 tablespoons shelled sunflower seeds
- 1 tablespoon polenta
- 1 tablespoon ground flax seeds
- 1 teaspoon all-purpose flour, or as needed
- ½ teaspoon cornmeal, or as needed
- 1 ¾ teaspoons salt
- 1 ½ teaspoon honey

Instructions

1. In a large mixing bowl, combine 1 cup warm water, 1/2 cup all-purpose flour, 1/2 cup whole wheat flour, 1/4 cup rye flour, and yeast. Cover the bowl with plastic wrap and set aside for five to six hours, or until the sponge bubbles and doubles in volume.
2. With a wooden spoon, stir 1 cup all-purpose flour, 1 cup whole wheat flour, 1/2 cup water, sunflower seeds, polenta, flax seeds, salt, and honey into a sponge until sticky dough ball forms, about three minutes. Scrape down the sides of the basin, cover with plastic wrap, and set aside for ten hours to overnight to double in volume. Using parchment paper, line a baking sheet. 1/2 teaspoon all-purpose flour and cornmeal on parchment paper
3. Scrape the dough from the bowl onto a lightly floured work surface, pressing down to remove any air bubbles and shaping it into a smooth oval loaf. Place the dough on the baking sheet that has been prepared. Dust the top of the loaf gently with flour, cover with plastic wrap, and let rise for one and half hours or until doubled in size.
4. Preheat the oven to 450 degrees Fahrenheit. On the bottom rack of the oven, place a baking dish filled with water.
5. Remove the plastic wrap from the rising dough and spritz the top with water.
6. Bake for thirty to thirty-five minutes in a preheated oven, sprinkle the top of the bread with water every eight to ten minutes, until brown and hollow when tapped. Place the bread on a wire rack to cool completely before slicing.

PIZZA BREAD

Preparation: 10 Minutes

Cook: 25 Minutes

Servings: 15

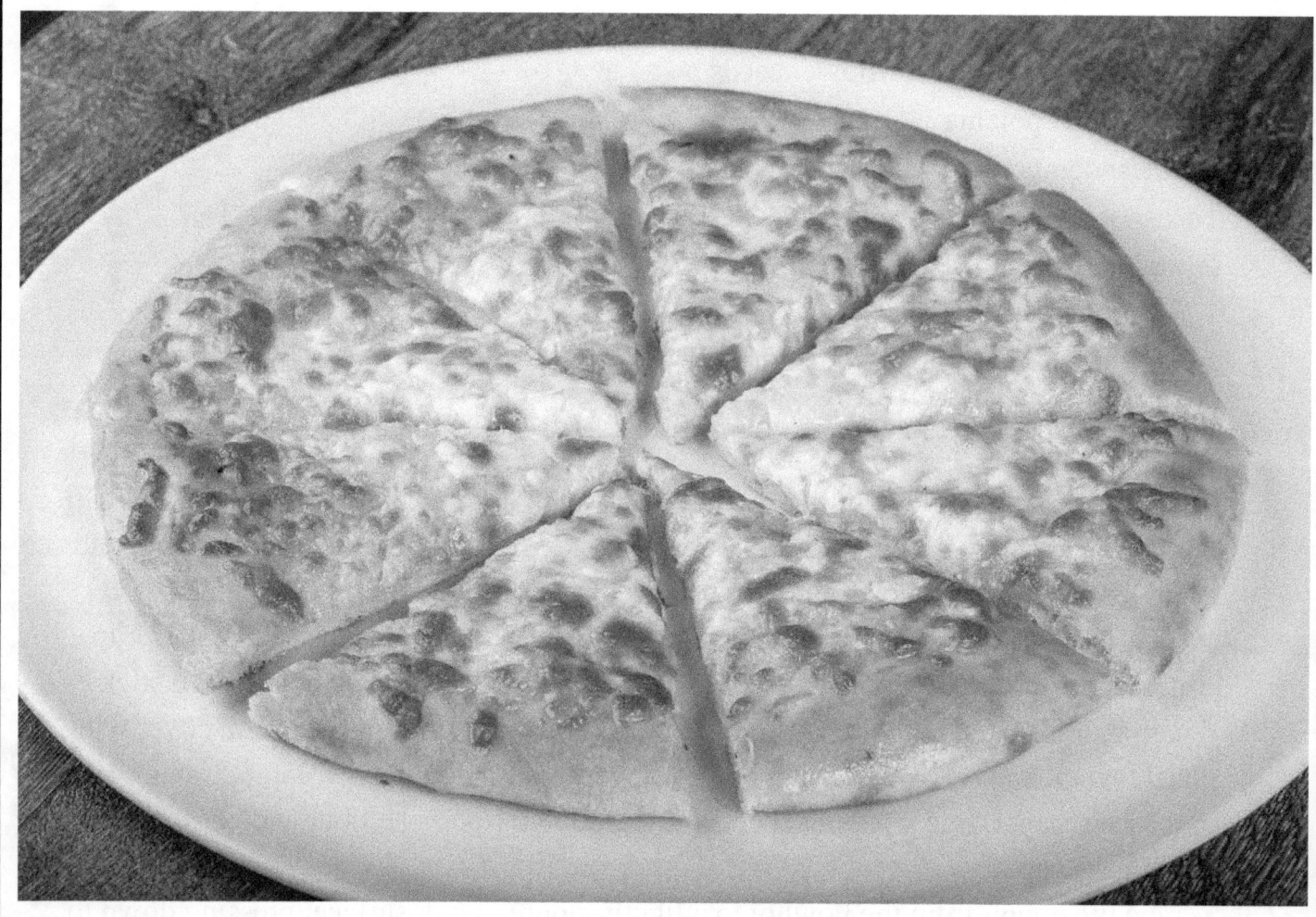

This simple recipe only requires a few basic ingredients and patting the dough onto the pan. With this method, there's no need to wait for the dough to rise.

Nutrition

Calories: 112 | Protein: 2.8g | Fat: 2.1g | Sodium: 156.2mg | Carbohydrates: 20.1g

Ingredients

1. 2 tablespoons vegetable oil
2. 1 cup warm water
3. 3 cups all-purpose flour
4. 1 package active dry yeast
5. 1 tablespoon white sugar
6. 1 teaspoon salt

Instructions

1. In a large mixing bowl, combine flour, salt, sugar, and yeast. Combine the oil and warm water in a mixing bowl. On a big pizza pan, spread out the ingredients. As desired, garnish.
2. Preheat oven to 375°F and bake for twenty to twenty-five minutes.

GLUTEN-FREE CHEESE AND HERB PIZZA CRUST

Preparation: 15 Minutes

Cook: 30 Minutes

Servings: 8

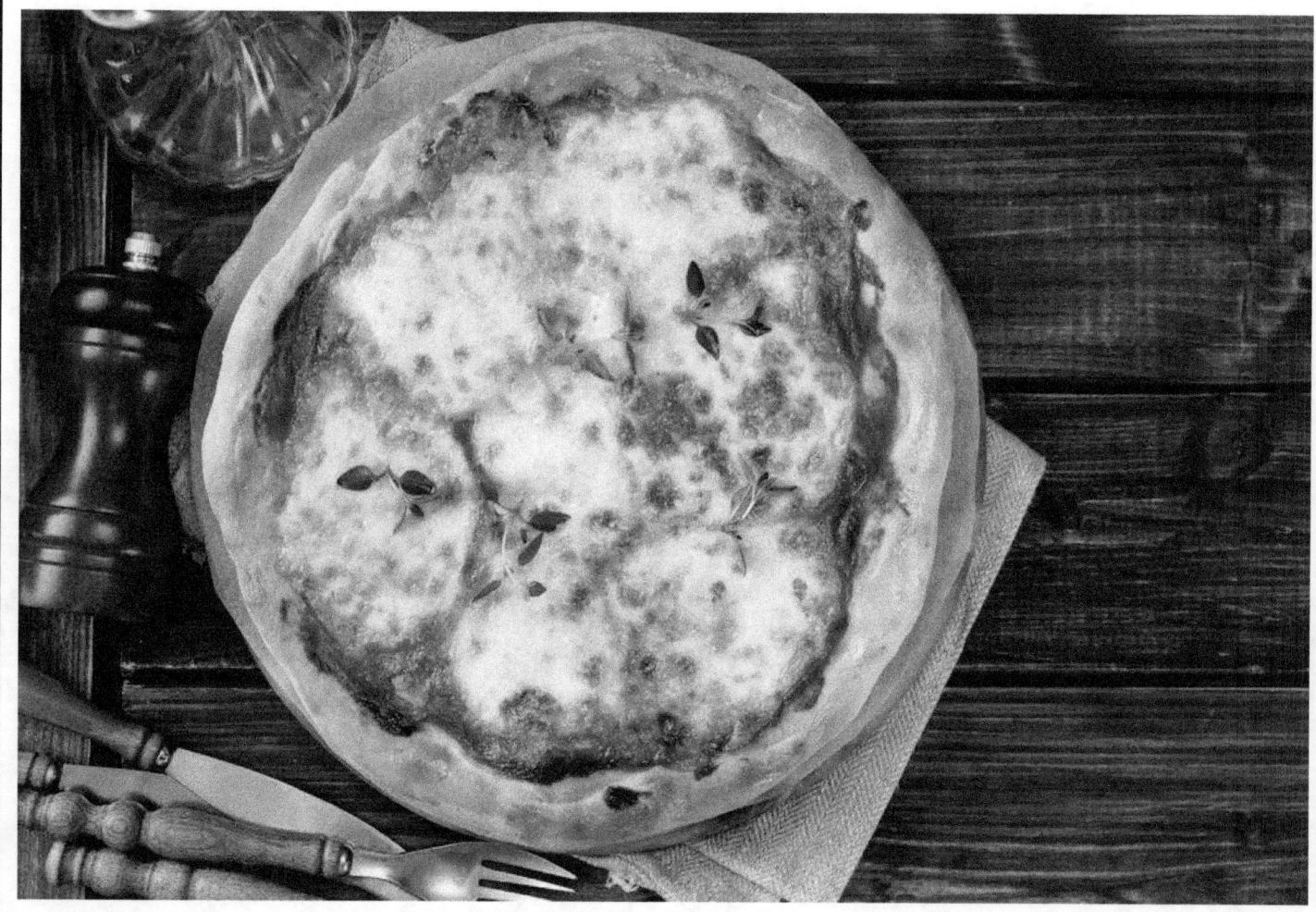

This is a gluten-free pizza crust version; it was discovered that baking it for 10 minutes before topping improves the texture.

Nutrition

Calories: 79 | Protein: 2.7g | Cholesterol: 25.5mg | Sodium: 300.3mg

Carbohydrates: 11.7g | Fat: 2.5g

Ingredients

- 1 egg
- ¼ cup grated Parmesan cheese
- 1 ½ teaspoon olive oil
- ¾ cup gluten-free all-purpose baking flour
- ½ teaspoon apple cider vinegar
- 1 cup lukewarm water
- 1 package active dry yeast
- ¼ cup garbanzo bean flour
- 1 teaspoon dried oregano
- 1 ½ teaspoons baking powder
- ½ teaspoon salt
- 1 teaspoon white sugar
- 1 teaspoon white sugar
- 1 teaspoon xanthan gum
- 1 teaspoon Italian seasoning
- ½ teaspoon minced garlic
- ¼ cup cornstarch
- ¼ cup tapioca starch

Instructions

1. Preheat the oven to 425 degrees Fahrenheit. Using cooking spray, grease a 15-inch pizza pan.
2. In a mixing bowl, whisk together all-purpose baking flour, garbanzo bean flour, cornstarch, tapioca starch, Parmesan cheese, baking powder, xanthan gum, Italian seasoning, oregano, and salt.
3. Dissolve 1 teaspoon white sugar in a small bowl of lukewarm water. Sprinkle yeast on top and set aside for three to five minutes, or until frothy.
4. In a separate bowl, whisk together the egg, olive oil, vinegar, 1 teaspoon sugar, and garlic until completely smooth. Whisk the yeast mixture into the egg mixture, then stir in the flour mixture until there are no dry lumps. Fill the prepared pan with dough, leaving the outer edge somewhat thicker than the middle.
5. Cook for ten to twelve minutes in a preheated oven until the dough has risen and firmed slightly.
6. Continue baking at 425 degrees F until the crust is golden brown, twenty to thirty minutes after adding your favorite toppings. Remove the pizza from the pan and place it straight on the oven rack for five minutes to crisp up the crust.

WHOLE WHEAT AND HONEY PIZZA DOUGH

Preparation: 10 Minutes

Cook: 10 Minutes

Servings: 12

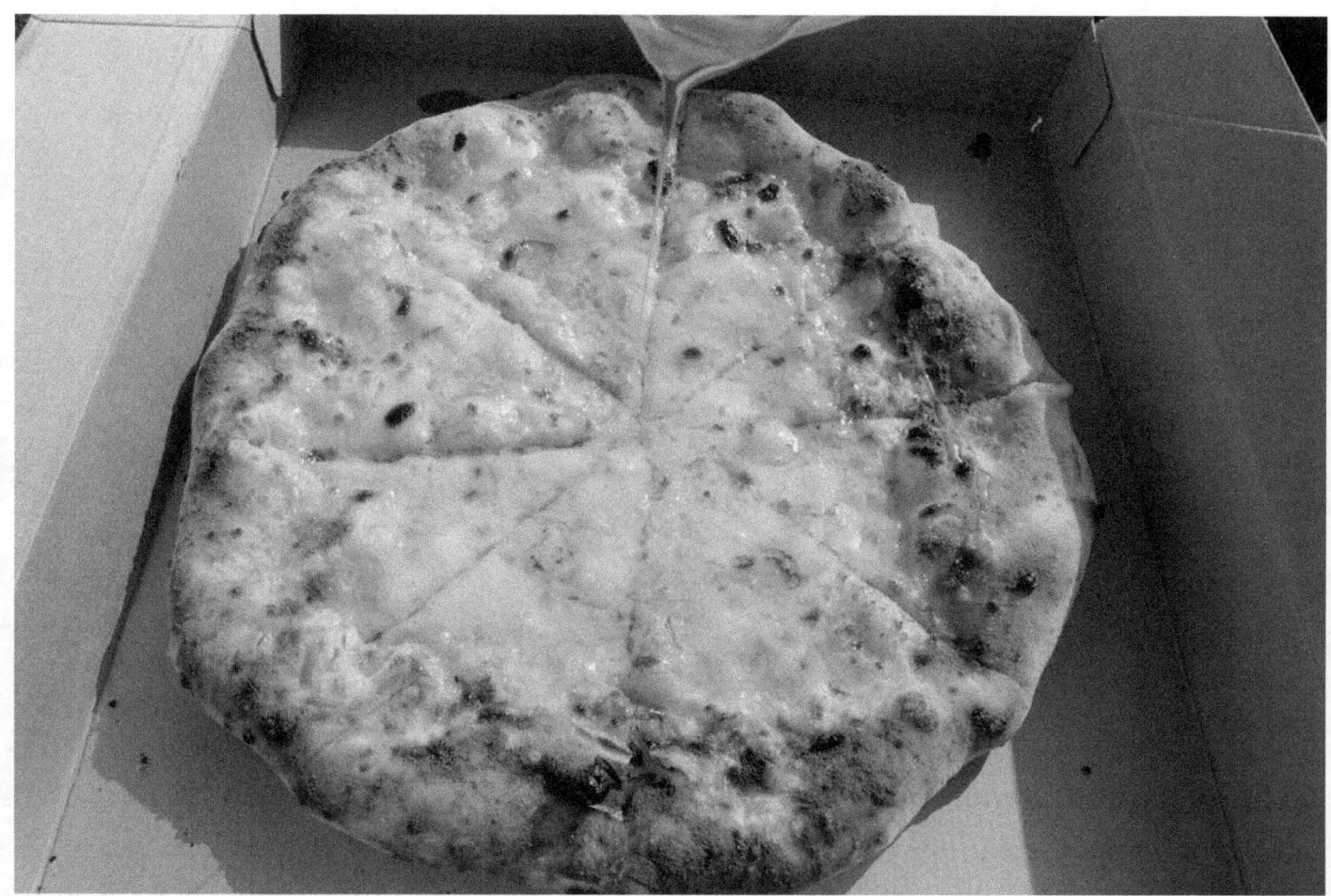

Quick, quick, and delicious homemade pizza dough that you can top however you like. This recipe yields a thin crust, but it may easily be doubled to make a thick crust.

Nutrition

Calories: 84 | Protein: 3.5g | Fat: 0.6g | Sodium: 196mg | Carbohydrates: 17.4g

Ingredients

- 2 cups whole wheat flour
- ¼ cup wheat germ
- 1 teaspoon salt
- 1 package active dry yeast
- 1 tablespoon honey
- 1 cup warm water

Instructions

1. Preheat the oven to 350 degrees Fahrenheit.
2. Dissolve yeast in warm water in a small dish. Allow ten minutes for the mixture to become creamy.
3. Combine flour, wheat germ, and salt in a large bowl and mix. In the center, make a well and pour in the honey and yeast mixture. To blend, stir everything together thoroughly. Cover and place in a warm place for a few minutes to rise.
4. Poke a few holes in the dough with a fork and roll it out on a floured pizza pan.
5. Bake for five to ten minutes, or until desired crispiness is attained, in a preheated oven.

AMAZING WHOLE WHEAT PIZZA CRUST

Preparation: 25 Minutes

Cook: 20 Minutes

Servings: 10

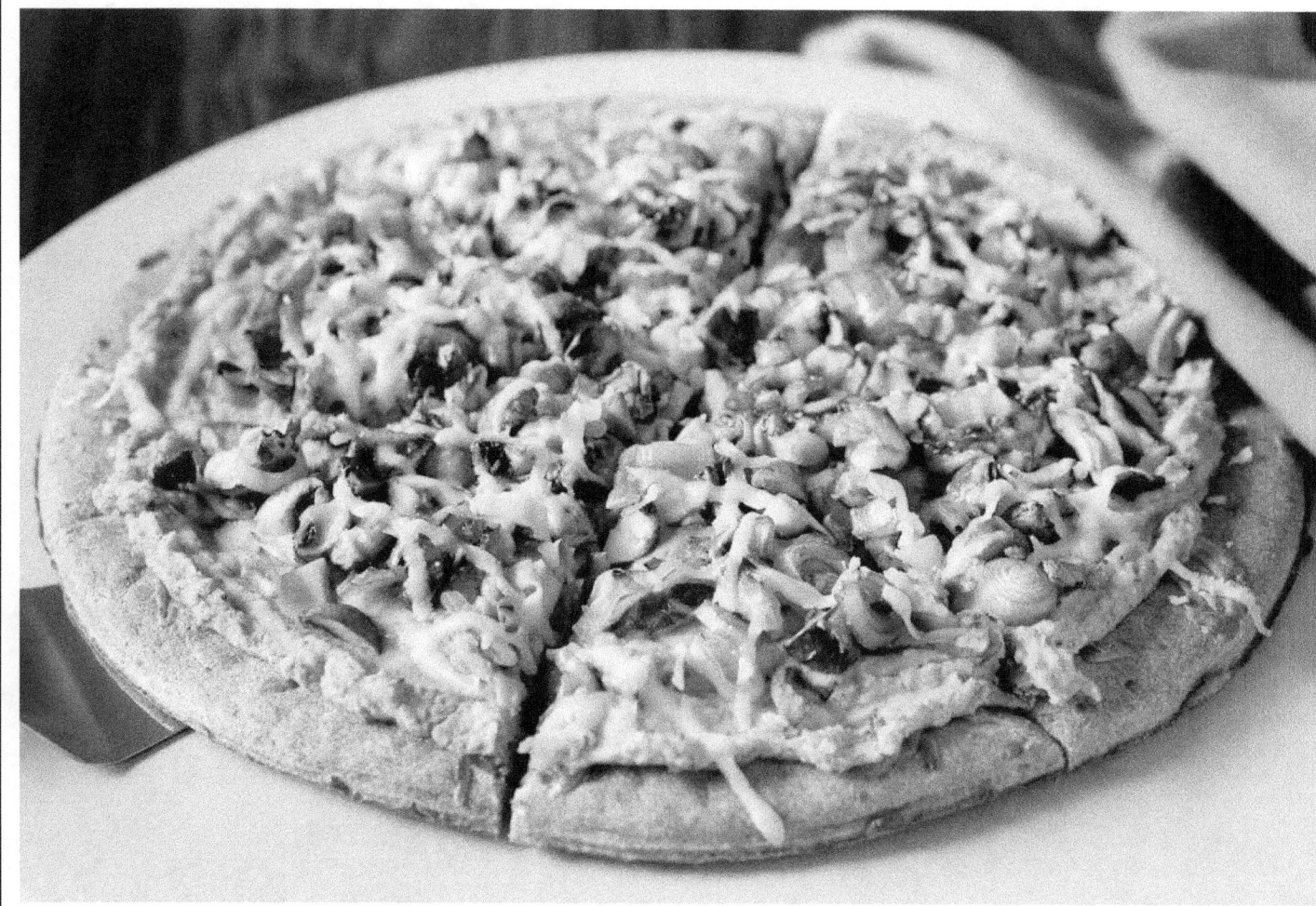

This whole wheat crust is soft and chewy on the inside and crisp on the outside. Toss with your favorite pizza toppings or make your pizza recipe.

Nutrition

Calories: 167 | Protein: 5.7g | Fat: 2g | Sodium: 235.8mg | Carbohydrates: 32.6g

Ingredients

- 2 cups whole wheat flour
- 1 package active dry yeast
- 1 cup warm water
- 1 teaspoon salt
- ¼ cup wheat germ
- 1 tablespoon honey

Instructions

1. Preheat the oven to 350 degrees Fahrenheit.
2. Dissolve yeast in warm water in a small bowl. Allow ten minutes for the mixture to become creamy.
3. Combine flour, wheat germ, and salt in a large mixing bowl. In the center, make a well and pour in the honey and yeast mixture. To blend, stir everything together thoroughly. Cover and place in a warm place for a few minutes to rise.
4. Poke a few holes in the dough with a fork and roll it out on a floured pizza pan.

VALENTINO'S PIZZA CRUST

Preparation: 5 Minutes

Cook: 2 Hours

Servings: 10

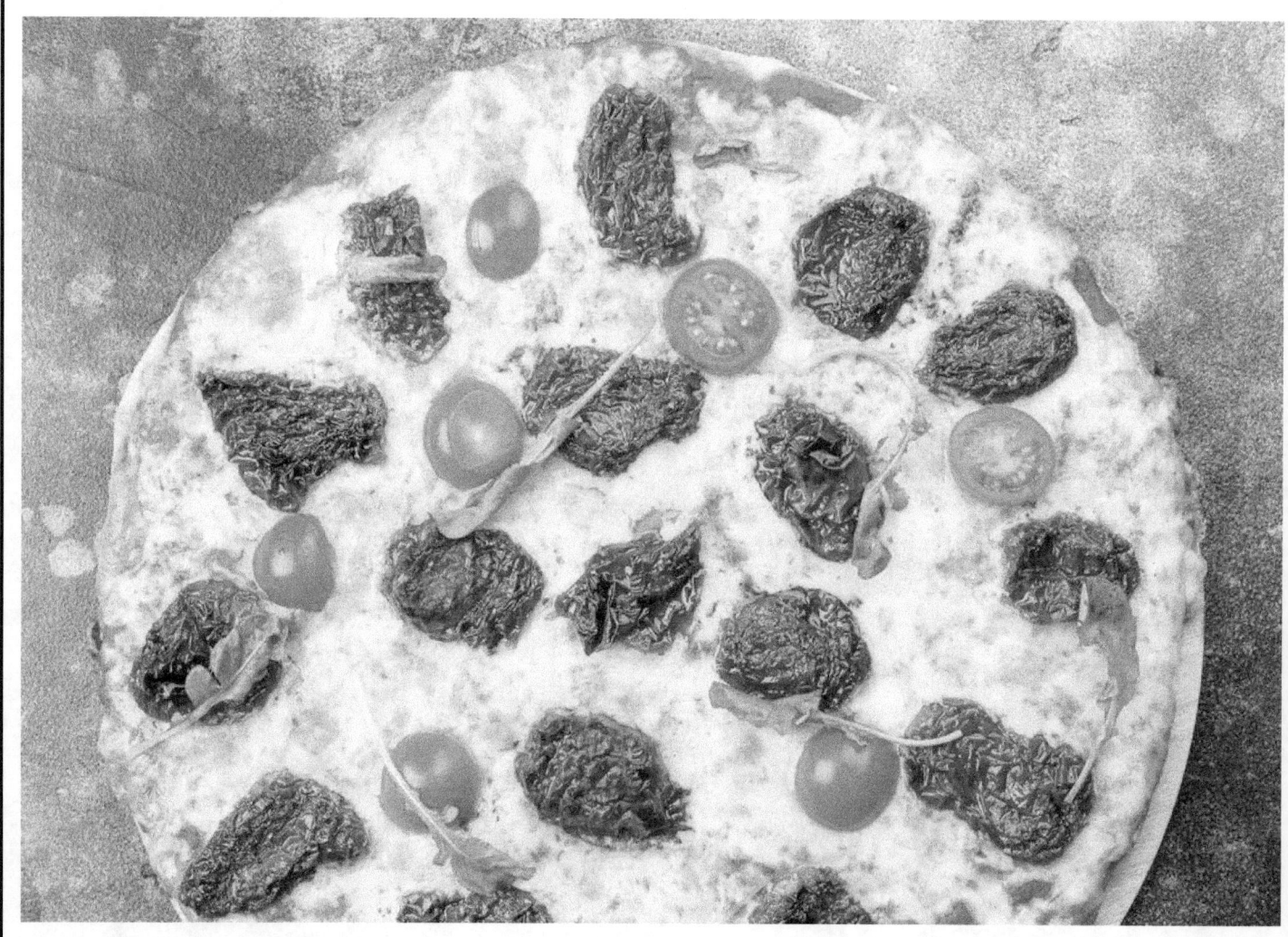

This pizza crust recipe is fantastic. We've discovered that baking it on a pizza stone makes it taste even better.

Nutrition

Calories: 21 | Protein: 0.4g | Carbohydrates: 1.8g | Cholesterol: 0.1mg

Sodium: 121mg | Fat: 1.4g

Ingredients

- 2 ½ cups all-purpose flour
- 3 tablespoons olive oil
- 1 teaspoon salt
- 1 cup warm water
- 2 ¼ teaspoons active dry yeast
- 1 tablespoon white sugar

Instructions

1. Stir together the water, sugar, and yeast until they are completely dissolved. Combine the olive oil and salt in a mixing bowl. Stir in the flour until it's completely mixed. Allow 10 minutes for the dough to rest.
2. Using olive oil-dipped fingertips, pat dough into pan or onto the pizza stone. Sprinkle basil, thyme, or other seasonings on the crust if preferred. In a preheated 425 degrees oven, top with your favorite pizza toppings and bake for fifteen to twenty minutes.

GRILL DOUGH

Preparation: 5 Minutes

Cook: 2 Hours

Servings: 12

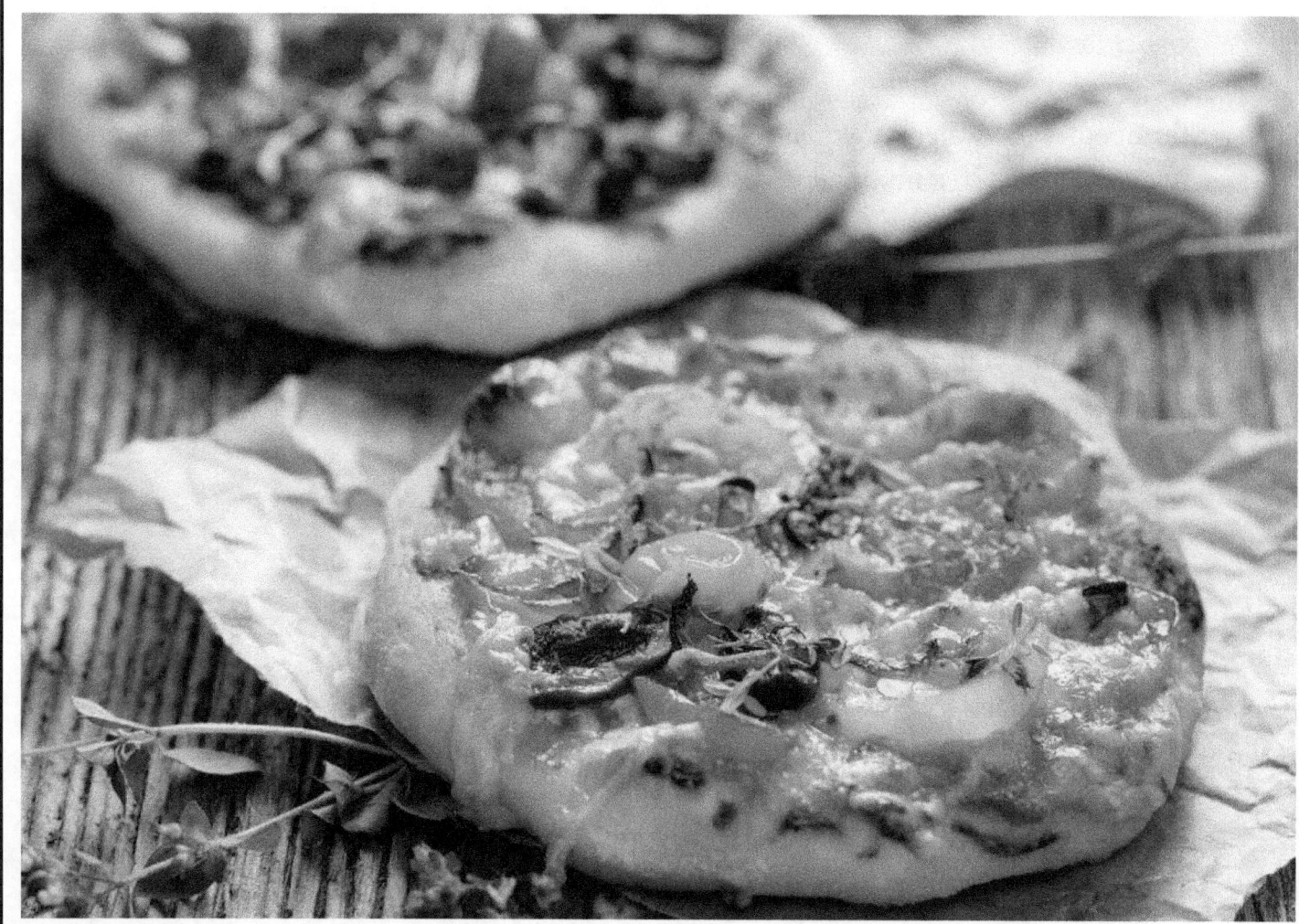

Especially nice in the summer. It can be assembled with desired toppings and cooked directly on the grill! If you like, you can make this recipe with whole wheat flour.

Nutrition

Calories: 93 | Protein: 2.5g | Fat: 1.4g | Sodium: 98.1mg | Carbohydrates: 17.3g

Ingredients

- ¾ cup warm water
- 1 tablespoon olive oil
- 2 tablespoons cornmeal for dusting
- 2 cups all-purpose flour
- ½ teaspoon salt
- ½ teaspoon white sugar
- 1 package active dry yeast

Instructions

1. Warm water is used to proof yeast.
2. Combine flour, salt, sugar, and oil in a separate bowl. In the center, make a well and pour in the yeast/warm water combination. In a large mixing bowl, thoroughly combine the ingredients until they form an elastic ball. Allow one and half hours for the cake to rise.
3. Roll out 1/2 of the dough on a floured surface. Cornmeal must be rubbed on the surface. Toppings of your choice can be sprinkled on top.
4. Spray grill with cooking spray. Grill dough for about five minutes or until toppings is melted. Rep with the second dough piece.

NO-YEAST PIZZA CRUST

Preparation: 15 Minutes

Cook: 10 Minutes

Servings: 8

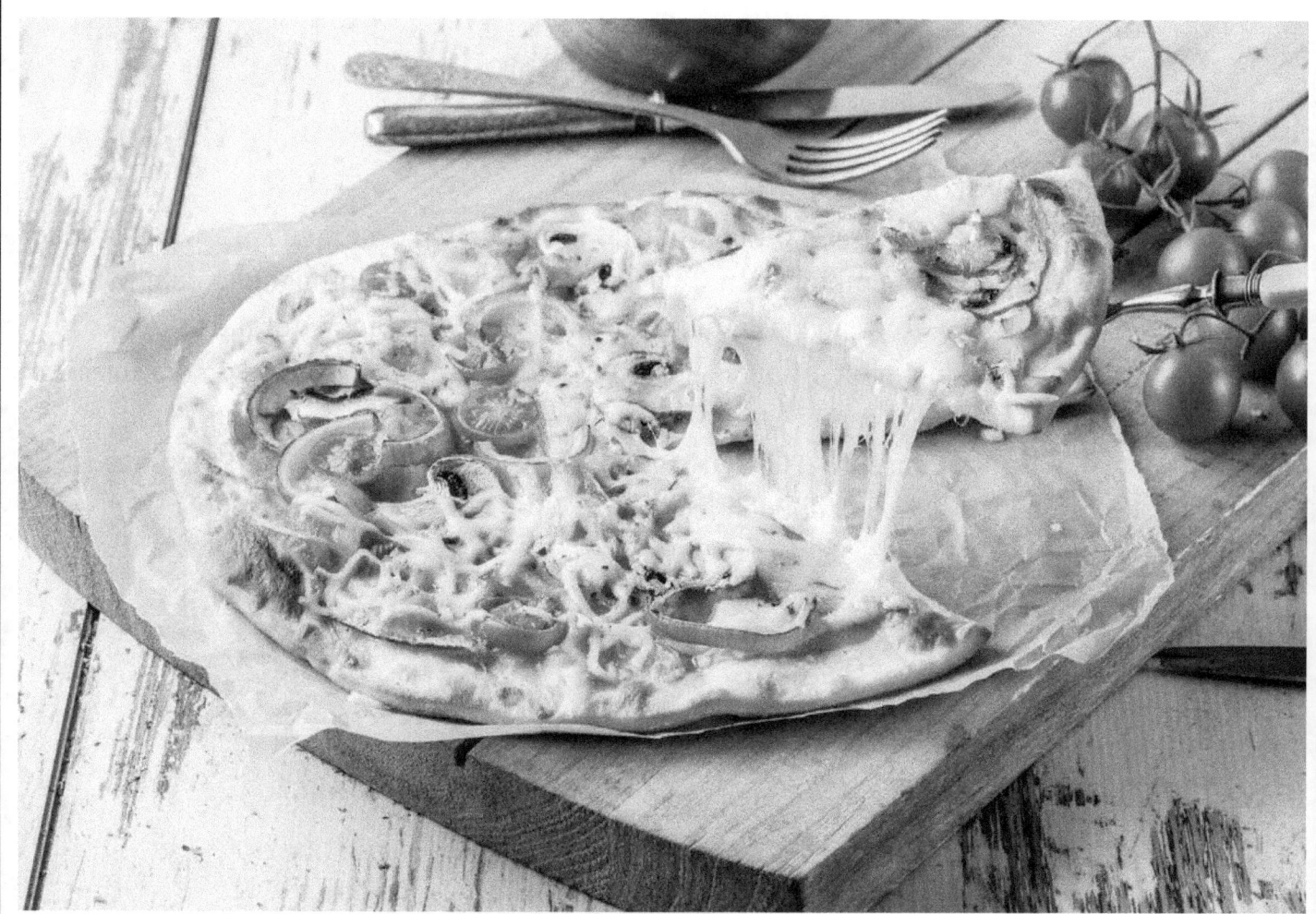

A delicious, quick pizza crust that doesn't require yeast.

Nutrition

Calories: 112 | Protein: 2.8g | Cholesterol: 0.3mg | Sodium: 215.8mg

Carbohydrates: 16.9g | Fat: 3.6g

Ingredients

- ½ cup fat-free milk
- 1 teaspoon baking powder
- 2 tablespoons olive oil
- 1 ⅓ cups all-purpose flour
- ½ teaspoon salt

Instructions

1. In a large bowl, combine flour, baking powder, and salt; stir in milk and olive oil until a soft dough form. Knead the dough ten times on a lightly floured board. Form a ball out of the dough. Allow dough to rest for ten minutes under an inverted bowl.
2. On a baking sheet, roll out the dough into a 12-inch circle.

COLLEEN'S POTATO CRESCENT ROLLS

Preparation: 30 Minutes

Cook: 30 Minutes

Servings: 32

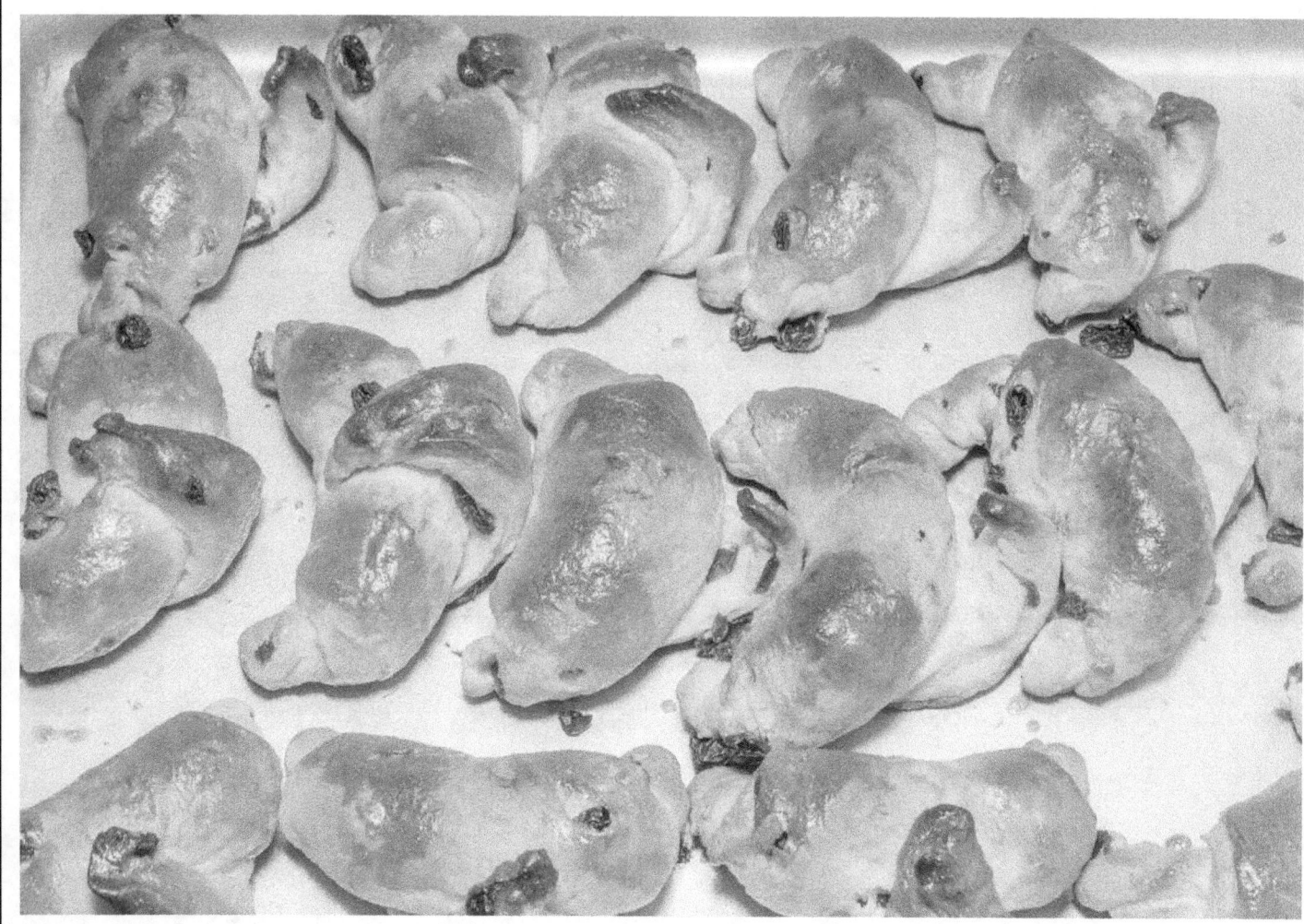

Every weekend, there are demands for these rolls from family, friends, and coworkers. They have fantastic taste! To add diversity to the butter topping, add garlic or cinnamon.

Nutrition

Calories: 140 | Protein: 3.3g | Cholesterol: 15.4mg | Sodium: 125.1mg

Carbohydrates: 26g | Fat: 6.3g

Ingredients

- 2 eggs
- 6 ½ cups all-purpose flour
- 2 potatoes, peeled and cut into 1-inch cubes
- 1 package active dry yeast
- ¼ cup butter, melted
- ⅔ cup shortening
- 1 ½ cups warm water
- 1 ½ teaspoons salt
- ⅔ cup white sugar

Instructions

1. Fill a saucepan halfway with water and add the potatoes. Bring to a boil, then reduce to low heat and cook until the vegetables are soft, about fifteen minutes. Drain, cool, and mash the potatoes.
2. Dissolve yeast in warm water in a large mixing dish. Allow ten minutes for the mixture to become creamy.
3. Mix in 1 cup mashed potatoes, sugar, shortening, eggs, salt, and 3 cups flour after the yeast is ready. 1/2 cup at a time, stir in the remaining flour until the dough is stiff but still flexible. Knead the dough on a lightly floured surface for about eight minutes, or until smooth and elastic. Lightly oil a large bowl then set the dough in it and turn it to coat it in oil. Refrigerate for at least eight hours and up to five days after covering with plastic wrap.
4. Turn the dough out onto a lightly floured surface to deflate it. Form the dough into rounds by dividing it into two equal parts. Each round should be rolled out to a 12-inch round. Brush each circle generously with melted butter and cut into 16 wedges. Starting with the large end, roll the wedges up tightly.
5. Place the points below and the ends twisted to make a crescent shape on lightly greased baking pans. Cover and set aside for one hour to rise. Preheat the oven to 400 degrees F in the meantime
6. Bake for fifteen to twenty minutes, or until golden brown, in a preheated oven.

POTATO BREAD RECIPE 2

Preparation: 5 Minutes

Cook: 3 Hours

Servings: 12

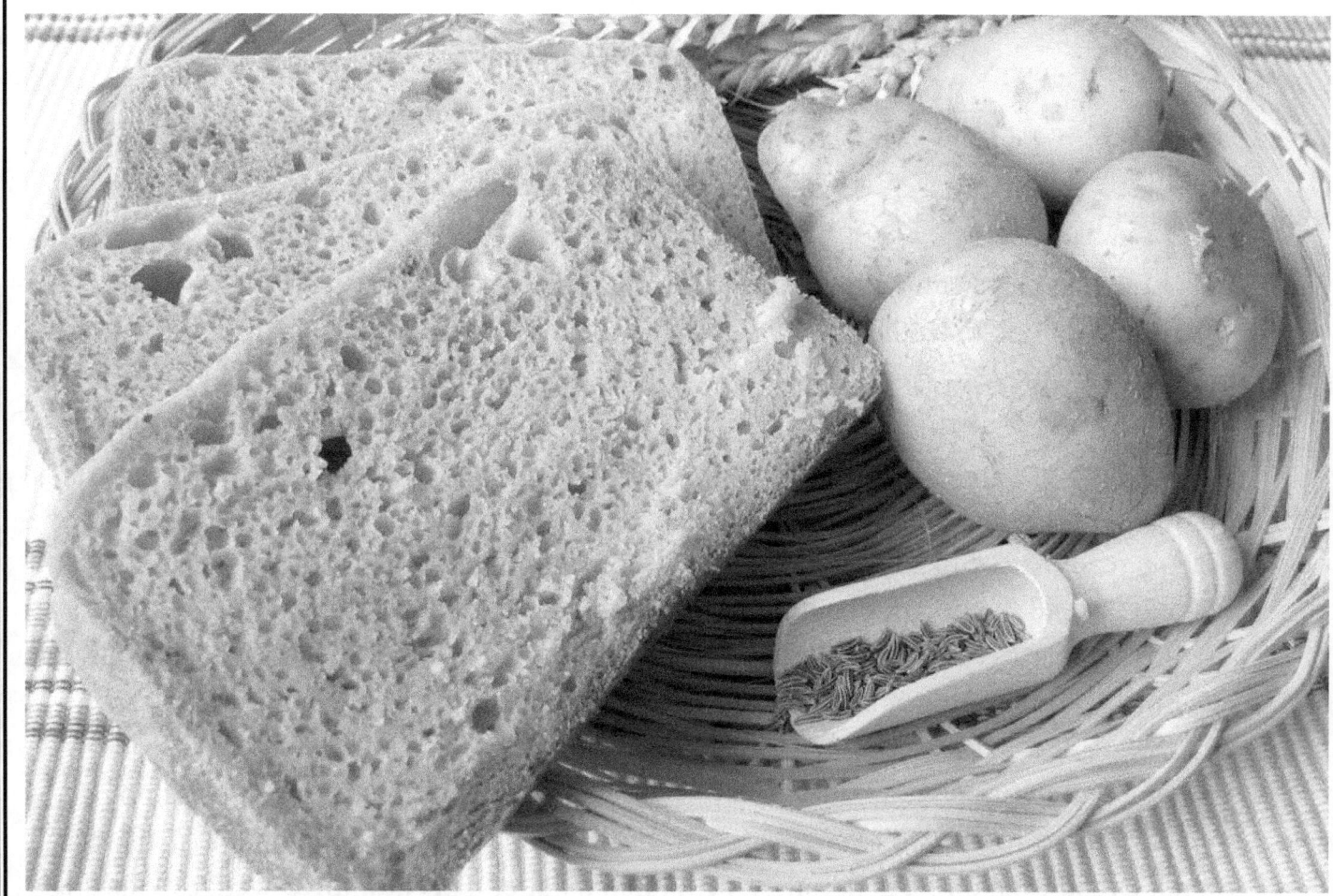

Excellent recipe. The texture is good. It's always proved to be a success with family and friends.

Nutrition

Calories: 42 | Protein: 0.8g | Cholesterol: 0.2mg | Sodium: 251.2mg

Carbohydrates: 4.6g | Fat: 2.3g

Ingredients

- 1 ⅓ cups warm water
- 2 tablespoons vegetable oil
- ½ cup dry potato flakes
- 2 tablespoons white sugar
- 1 ¾ teaspoon active dry yeast
- 3 ¼ cups bread flour
- 2 tablespoons dry milk powder
- 1 ¼ teaspoons salt

Instructions

Place the ingredients in the bread maker in the manufacturer's recommended order. Set the machine to the Light Crust setting.

CRUSTY POTATO BREAD

Preparation: 5 Minutes

Cook: 3 Hours

Servings: 15

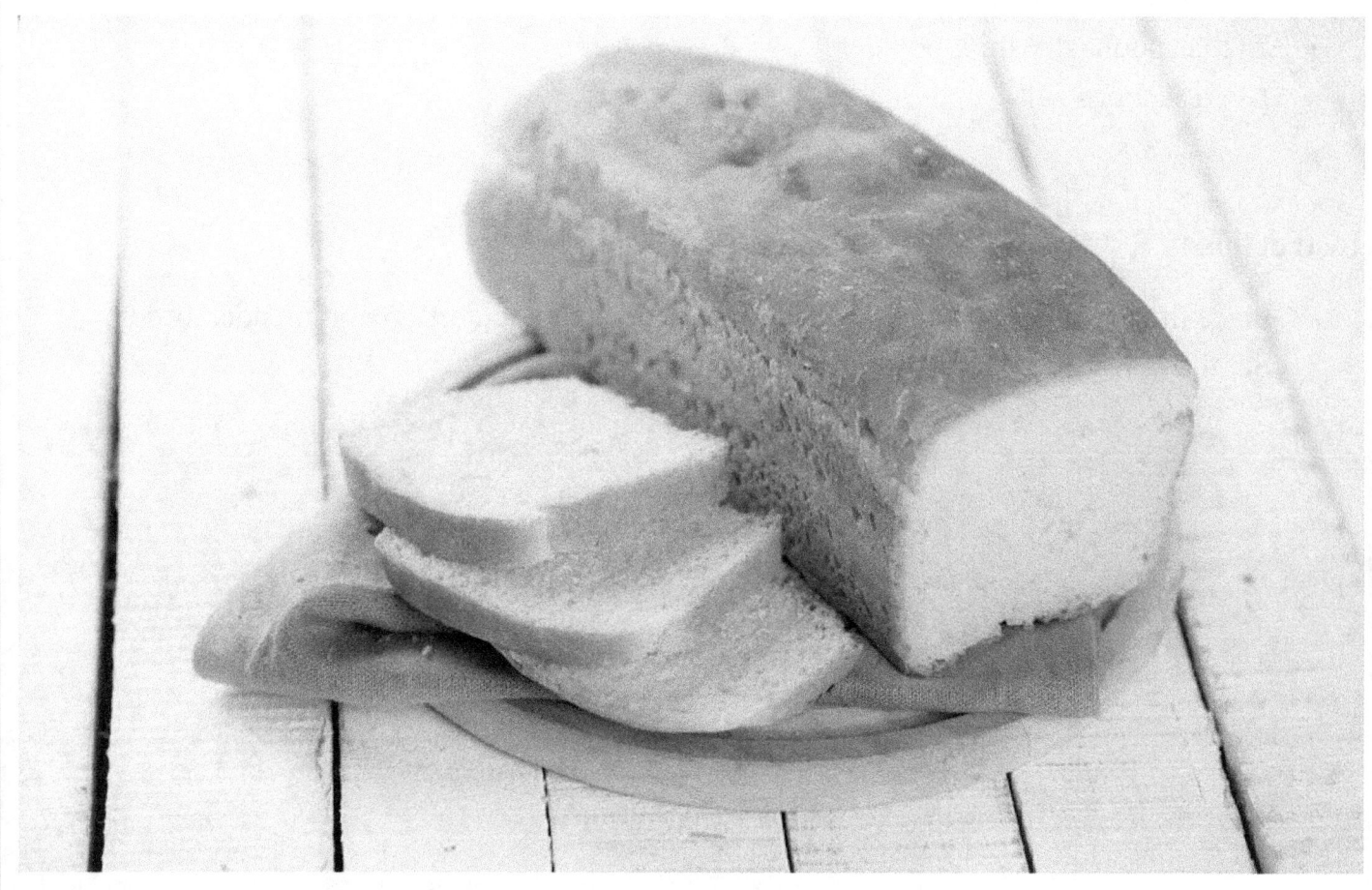

This hearty bread has a fantastic crust and a great flavor, and a delicious taste.

Nutrition

Calories: 24 | Protein: 0.3g | Cholesterol: 4.1mg | Sodium: 245.2mg

Carbohydrates: 2.2g | Fat: 1.6g

Ingredients

- 1 ¼ cups water
- 3 ¼ cups bread flour
- 2 teaspoons instant yeast
- 1 tablespoon white sugar
- 2 tablespoons butter
- ½ cup instant mashed potato flakes
- 1 ½ teaspoons salt

Instructions

Place the ingredients in the bread machine pan in the manufacturer's recommended order. Select the White Bread Cycle and press the Start button.

POTATO ROSEMARY BREAD

Preparation: 30 Minutes

Cook: 40 Minutes

Servings: 24

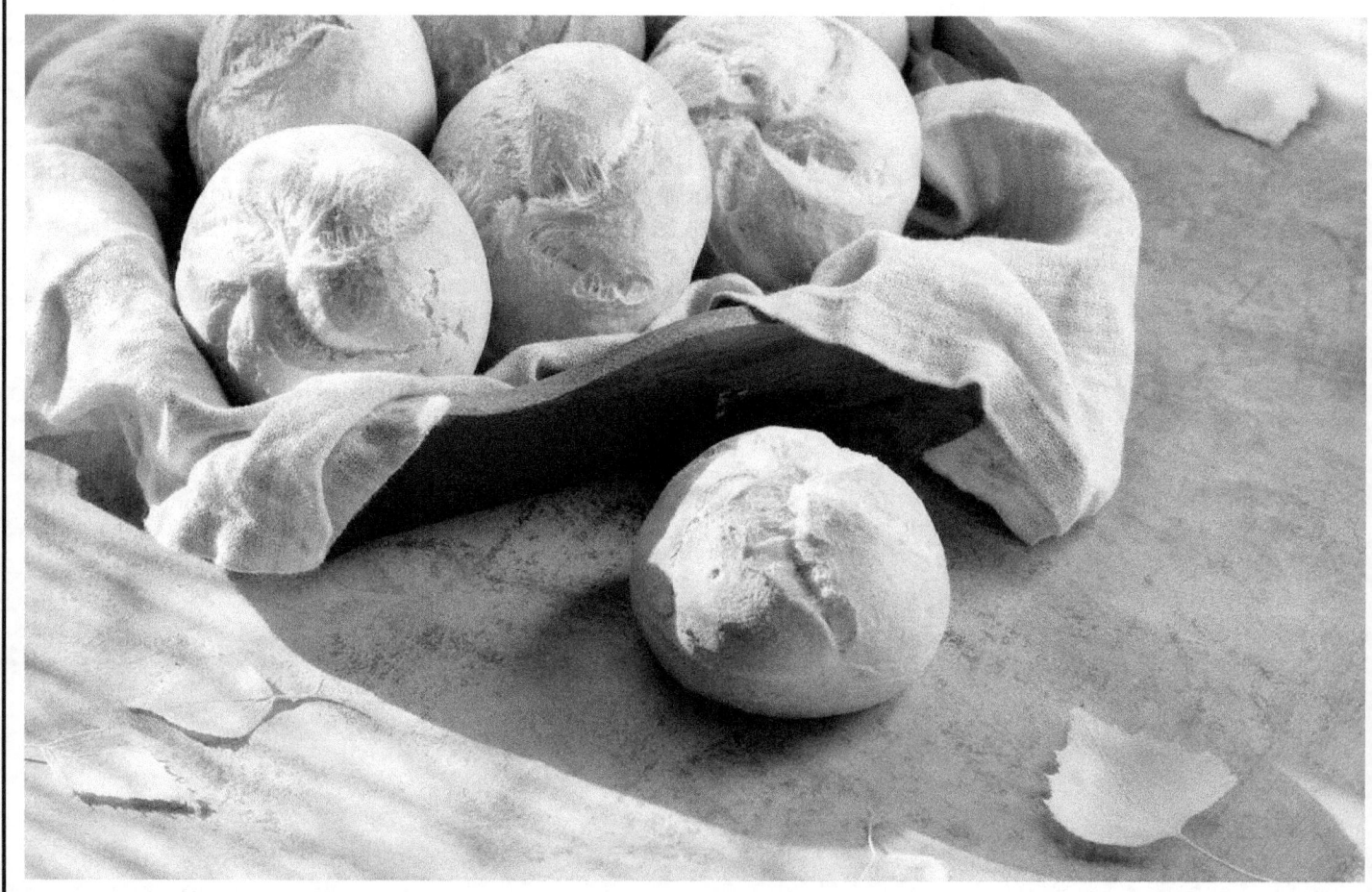

A rosemary-flavored potato bread that's simple to make.

Nutrition

Calories: 155 | Protein: 5g | Cholesterol: 17.9mg | Sodium: 529.3mg

Carbohydrates: 25.9g | Fat: 3.3g

Ingredients

- 1 egg, beaten
- ½ cup dry potato flakes
- 3 cups bread flour
- 1 ⅛ cups warm water
- 2 tablespoons olive oil
- 1 tablespoon cornmeal
- 1 teaspoon dried rosemary, crushed
- 1 ½ teaspoon bread machine yeast
- 2 tablespoons nonfat dry milk powder
- 1 tablespoon white sugar
- 2 teaspoons kosher salt
- 1 teaspoon salt

Instructions

1. In the sequence recommended by the manufacturer, measure and add warm water, olive oil, dry milk, potato flakes, sugar, rosemary, salt, bread flour, and yeast to your bread machine and select the Dough cycle and press the Start button.
2. Cut the dough into 12 equal pieces. Roll each into a 10-inch rope; coil the rope and tuck the end through the center. Place 2 inches apart on a cornmeal-dusted baking sheet. Allow forty-five minutes for the dough to rise.
3. Brush the tops with egg glaze or melted butter and kosher salt lightly. Bake for fifteen to twenty minutes at 375 degrees F.

CLARE'S WHOLE WHEAT POTATO BREAD

Preparation: 25 Minutes

Cook: 35 Minutes

Servings: 24

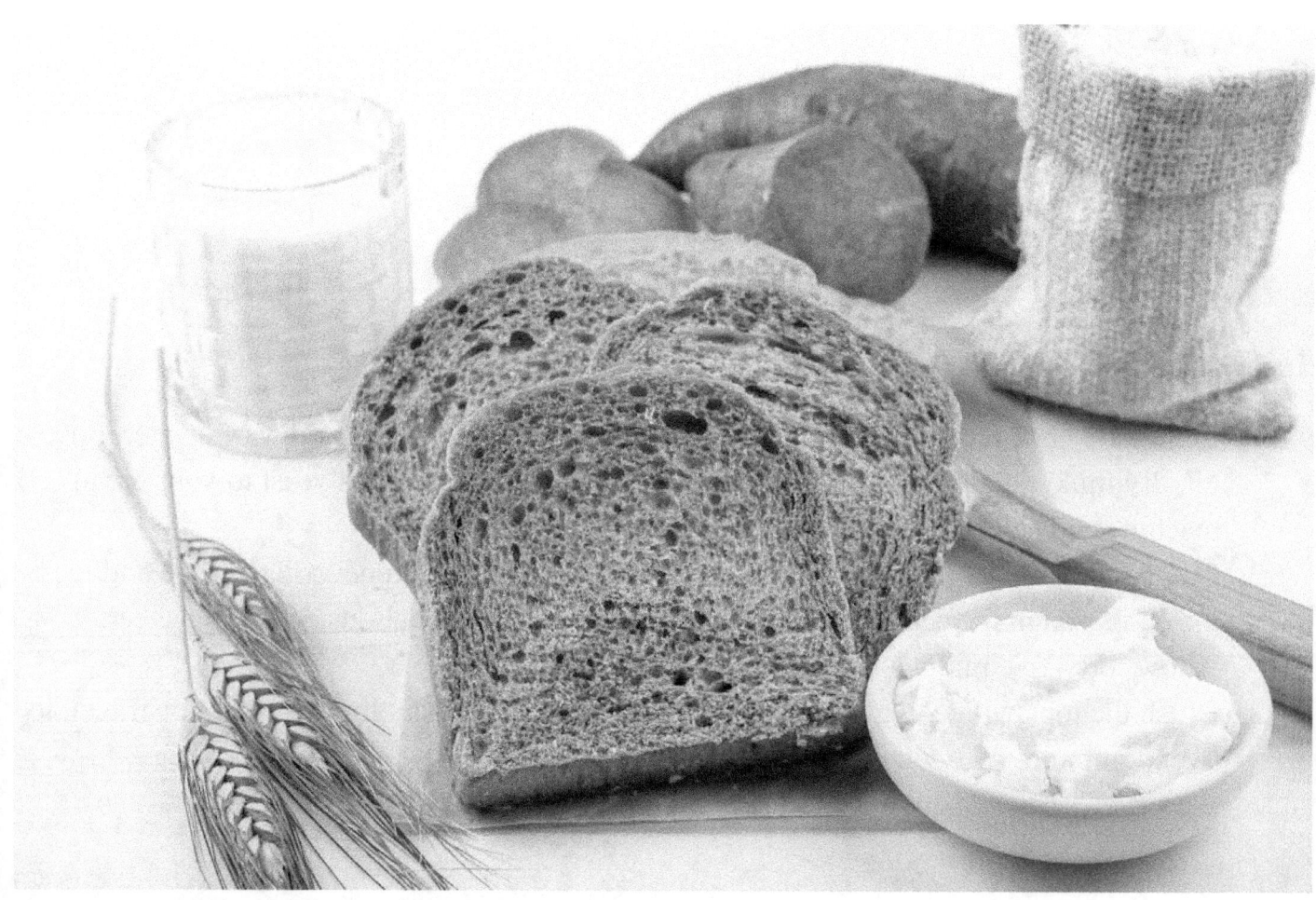

This is a recipe passed down through the ages. It is an ideal dish for any family.

Nutrition

Calories: 132 | Protein: 4.2g | Cholesterol: 16.5mg | Sodium: 280mg

Carbohydrates: 23.2g | Fat: 2.9g

Ingredients

- 2 eggs, beaten
- 1 ½ cups instant mashed potato flakes
- 2 ½ cups whole wheat flour
- 2 cups all-purpose flour
- 2 packages of active dry yeast
- ¼ cup honey
- 2 ½ teaspoons salt
- 1 ¼ cups warm milk
- 1 ½ cups warm water
- ¼ cup margarine

Instructions

1. Mix the all-purpose flour, potato flakes, salt, and yeast in a large mixing bowl. Combine the water, milk, margarine, honey, and eggs in a separate bowl. In a separate bowl, whisk together the liquid and dry ingredients. Gradually include whole wheat flour until the dough is evenly moistened. Knead five minutes Place in a greased mixing bowl, cover with a clean kitchen towel, and let rise for one hour or until doubled in size.
2. Two 5x9-inch loaf pans will be greased. Punch down the dough and form it into loaves before placing it in the pans. Allow one hour for the dough to rise in the pans.
3. Preheat the oven to 375 degrees Fahrenheit. Bake for thirty-five minutes, or until loaves are lightly browned and hollow when tapped.

ZADI'S POTATO BREAD

Preparation: 20 Minutes

Cook: 30 Minutes

Servings: 24

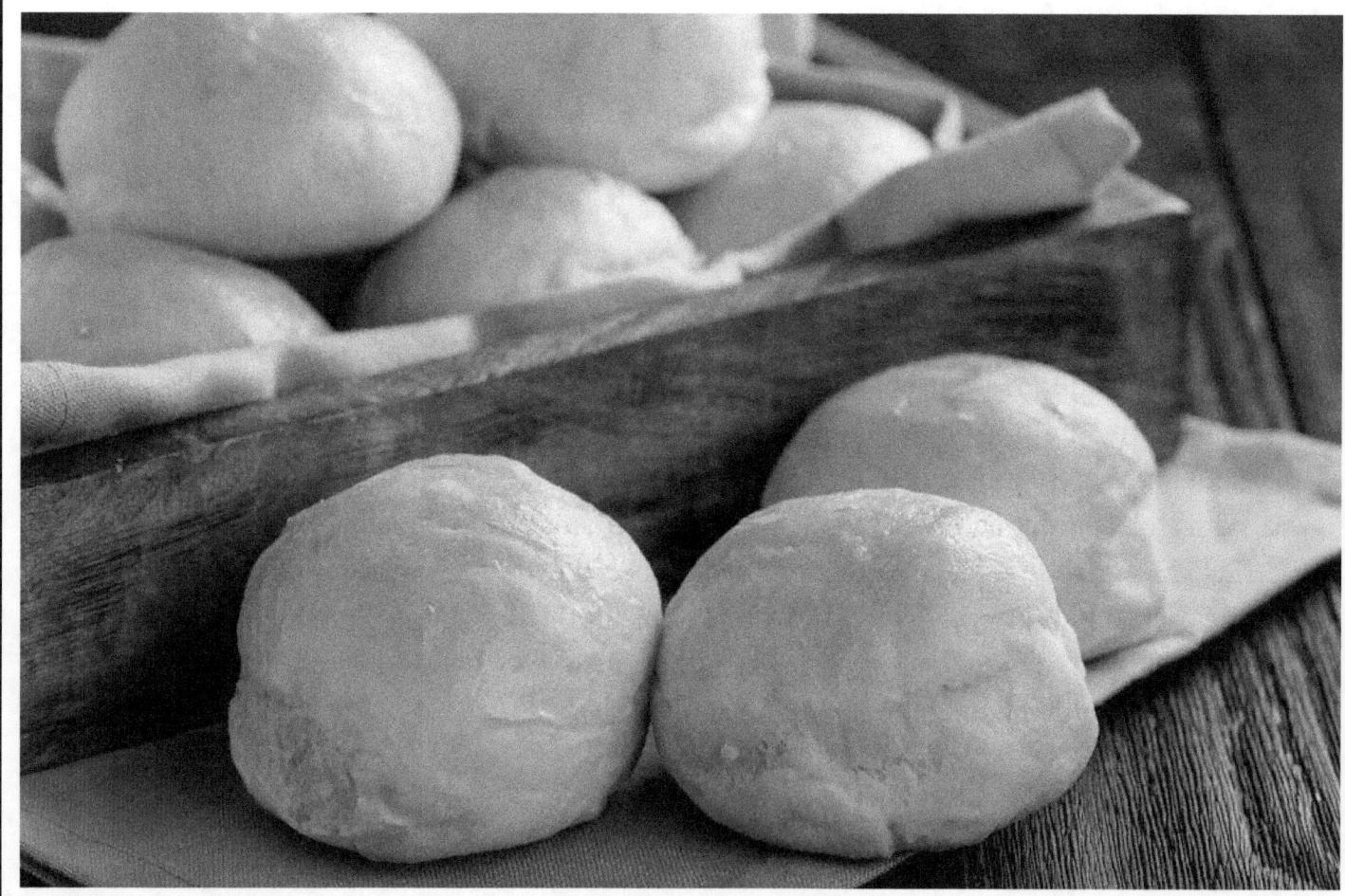

Instead of complete loaves of bread, this recipe can be used to produce rolls. This dish is perfect for any holiday dinner.

Nutrition

Calories: 47 | Protein: 0.8g | Fat: 2.7g | Cholesterol: 7.6mg | Sodium: 415.8mg

Carbohydrates: 5.2g

Ingredients

- 4 cups water
- 1 cup instant mashed potato flakes
- 2 packages of active dry yeast
- 10 cups bread flour, divided
- ¼ cup dry buttermilk powder
- ⅓ cup white sugar
- ⅓ cup butter
- 4 teaspoons salt

Instructions

1. In a saucepan over low heat, bring the water, butter, sugar, buttermilk powder, and salt to a simmer. Remove from the fire, stir thoroughly, and set aside to cool to between 105 to 110 degrees Fahrenheit. Sprinkle the yeast on top of the mixture. And set aside for about ten minutes or until creamy foam forms. Combine the instant mashed potato flakes with the remaining ingredients and stir thoroughly.
2. Pour the yeast mixture into the work bowl of a standing mixer fitted with a dough paddle, and gradually add 8 cups of bread flour, 1 cup at a time, to the liquid.
3. Knead the dough for about 8 minutes on a floured surface, adding the remaining flour to the dough as you knead. Form the dough into a ball and set it in a large greased bowl until smooth and elastic. Turn the dough over in the dish to coat the top, cover with a cloth. And let it rise for about one hour, or until doubled in size.
4. Spray 2 9x5 inch loaf pans with cooking spray. Punch down the dough, divide it in half, and form each half into a loaf. Place the loaves, seam sides down, in the baking pans, cover with a towel and let rise until doubled, about thirty minutes.
5. Preheat the oven to 350 degrees Fahrenheit
6. Bake for thirty minutes in a preheated oven or until the tops of the loaves is golden brown and hollow when tapped. Cool on a wire rack after removing from pans.

HIGH RISE DINNER ROLLS

Preparation: 30 Minutes

Cook: 25 Minutes

Servings: 9

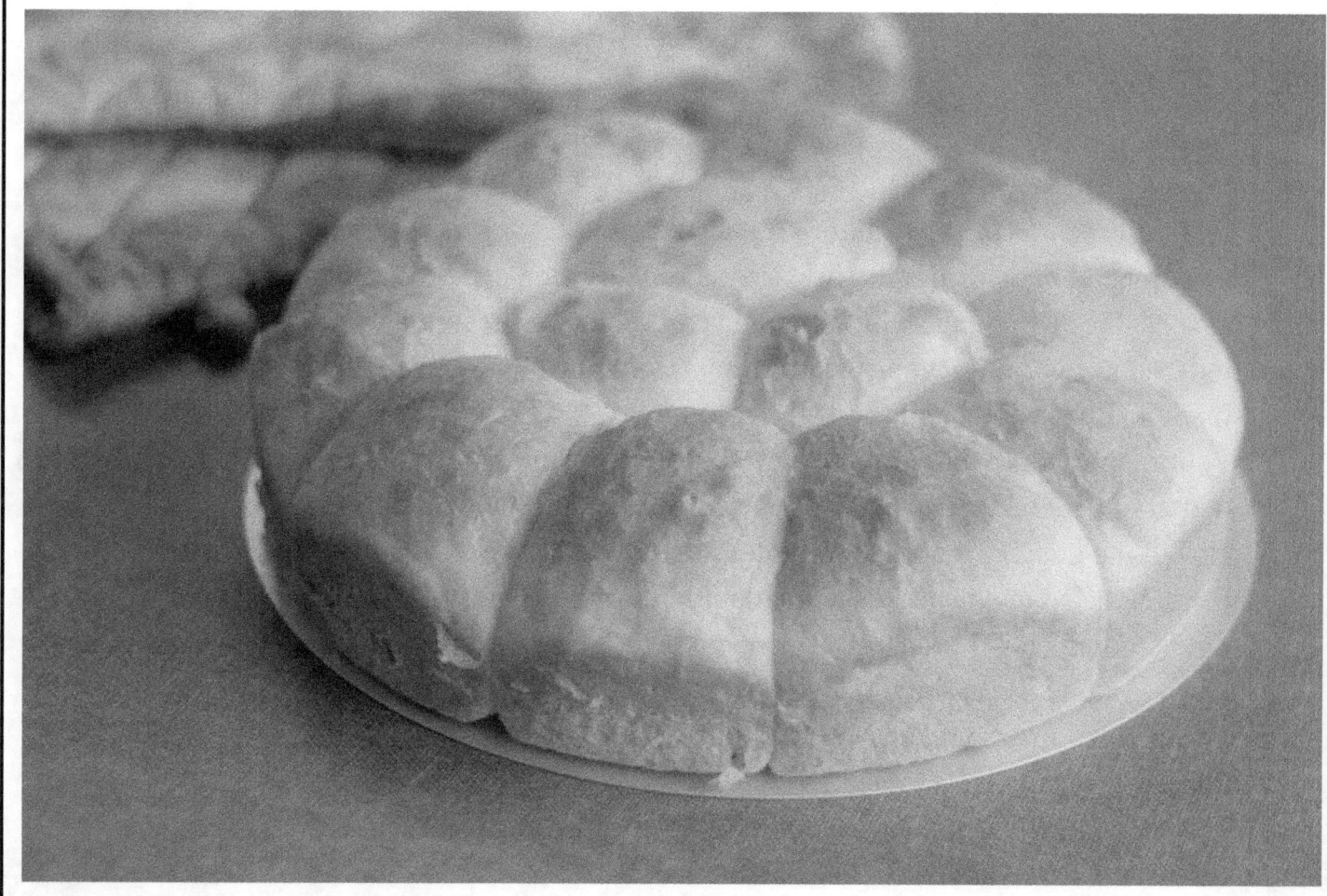

Pull-apart rolls with sensitive crusts that are soft and tall.

Nutrition

Calories: 252 | Protein: 6.9g | Cholesterol: 38.7mg | Sodium: 344.8mg

Carbohydrates: 38.9g | Fat: 8g

Ingredients

- 1 egg
- ½ cup instant mashed potato flakes
- 1 tablespoon white sugar
- 2 tablespoons white sugar   2 cups unbleached all-purpose flour
- 3 tablespoons butter, softened
- 1 teaspoon salt
- 1 cup warm buttermilk
- ¼ cup warm water
- ½ teaspoon vegetable oil, or as needed
- 2 tablespoons melted butter (or as needed), divided
- 1 cup whole wheat flour 1 package active dry yeast

Instructions

1. In a small bowl, dissolve 1 tablespoon sugar in warm water and sprinkle the yeast on top. The temperature of the water should not exceed 100 degrees Fahrenheit. Allow sitting for five minutes or until the yeast softens and forms a creamy foam. Turn the dough out onto a floured surface and knead for three minutes, or until smooth and elastic.
2. Form the dough into a ball, brush with vegetable oil, cover, and set aside to rise until doubled in size, about one hour.
3. Punch the dough down gently and divide it into 9 equal pieces. Make balls out of the pieces. Place the rolls in an 8x8-inch baking dish, slightly touching each other, and grease the dish. Melted butter will be brushed over the tops. Allow the rolls to rise in a warm location for thirty to forty-five minutes or until they have doubled in size. The rolls should rise above the pan's rim and be crammed in.
4. Preheat the oven to 400 degrees Fahrenheit. Bake the rolls for twenty-five to thirty minutes in a preheated oven until golden brown.
5. Brush the tops of the heated rolls with melted butter again, set aside to cool slightly before turning out of the pan and pulling apart. Warm the dish before serving.

HAWAIIAN SWEET BREAD

Preparation: 15 Minutes

Total: 15 Minutes

Servings: 15

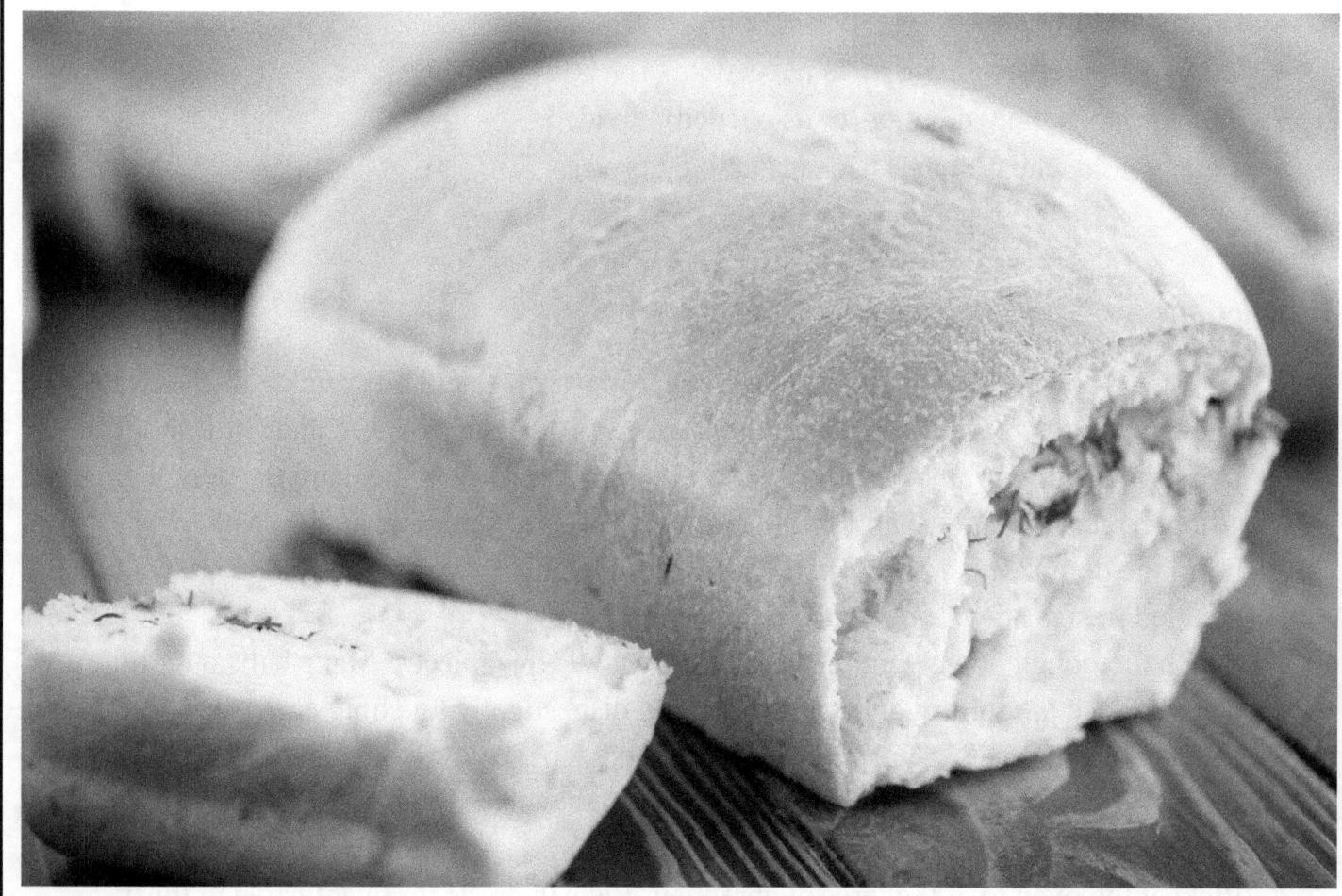

Flavorful, slightly sweet bread that's ideal for French toast and summer sandwiches on its own.

Nutrition

Calories: 116 | Protein: 3.8g | Cholesterol: 5.6mg | Sodium: 313.9mg

Carbohydrates: 18.4g | Fat: 2.8g

Ingredients

- 2 eggs
- 3 cups all-purpose flour
- 4 tablespoons margarine
- 1 cup warm water
- 5 tablespoons white sugar
- 2 tablespoons dry milk powder
- ¼ teaspoon vanilla extract
- 2 tablespoons dry milk powder
- 2 tablespoons dry potato flakes
- 2 tablespoons dry potato flakes
- ¾ teaspoon salt
- 1 tablespoon active dry yeast
- ¼ teaspoon lemon extract

Instructions

1. Measure the ingredients into the bread machine in the manufacturer's recommended order.
2. Set the machine to make dough.
3. In a 9x5 inch loaf pan, place the dough. Allow rising until it has doubled in size. Preheat the oven to 350°F
4. Preheat the oven to 350°F and bake for thirty minutes. When thumped, the crust should be brown, and the bread should sound hollow.

WHOLE WHEAT PUMPKIN BREAD

Preparation: 10 Minutes

Cook: 50 Minutes

Servings: 18

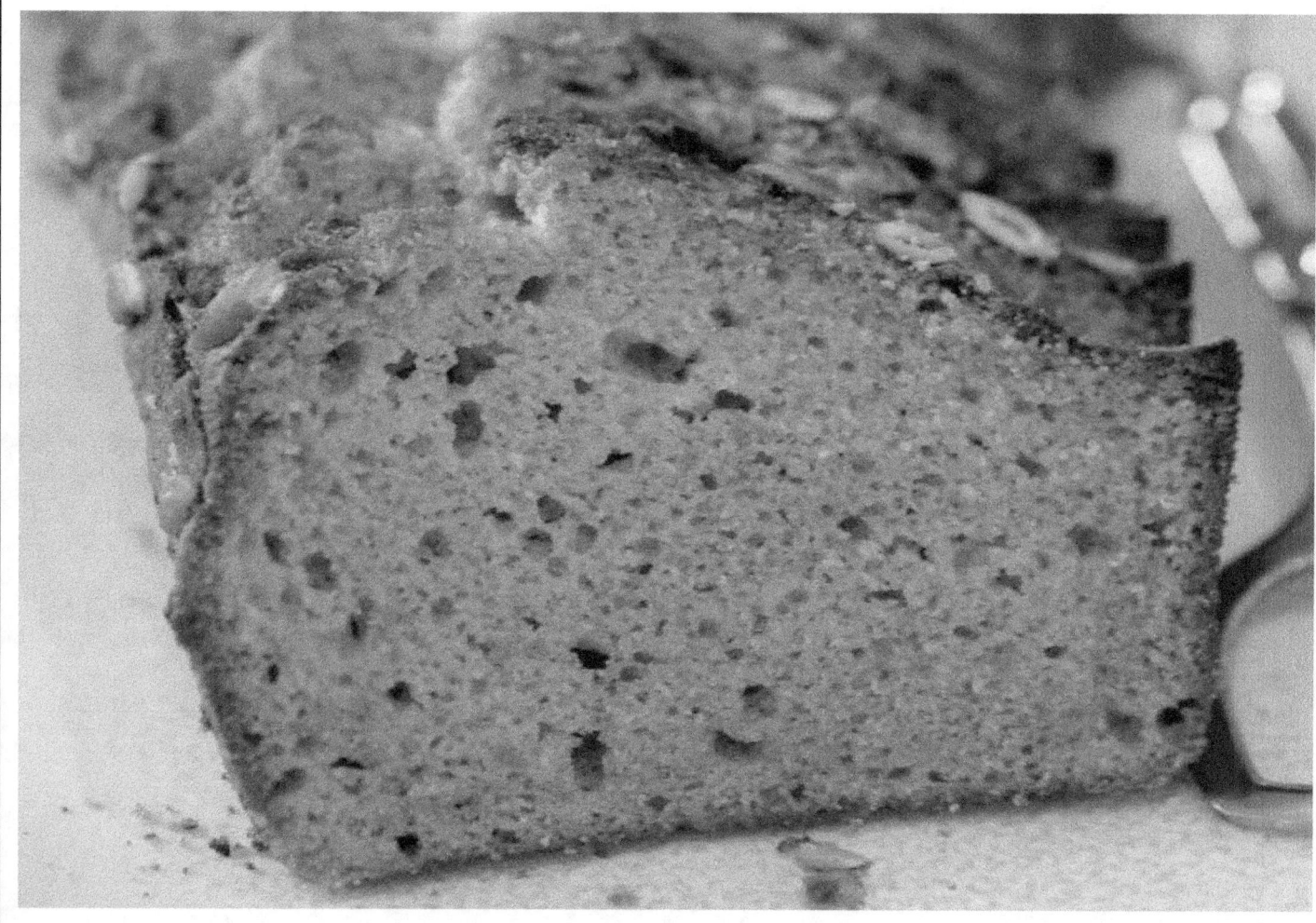

This soft and delicious bread is nicely spiced with cloves, cinnamon, nutmeg, and pumpkin. This recipe makes one loaf or 18 muffins.

Nutrition

Calories: 179 | Protein: 3.3g | Cholesterol: 18.2mg | Sodium: 188.9mg

Carbohydrates: 25.4g | Fat: 8.1g

Ingredients

- 2 eggs
- ½ cup raisins
- ¼ cup canola oil
- 1 cup whole wheat flour
- 1 cup pumpkin puree
- 1 cup coarsely chopped walnuts
- 1 cup white sugar
- ½ teaspoon ground nutmeg
- ⅔ cup all-purpose flour
- ½ teaspoon baking powder ½ teaspoon ground cloves
- 1 teaspoon ground cinnamon
- 1 teaspoon baking soda
- ½ teaspoon salt

Instructions

1. Preheat the oven to 375°F
2. Place the raisins in a bowl and cover with 1 inch of boiling water. Allow three to four minutes for raisins to plump up and rehydrate. Drain the raisins and set aside 1/3 cup of the soaking liquid in another dish.
3. In a large bowl, combine whole wheat flour, all-purpose flour, cinnamon, baking soda, baking powder, salt, cloves, and nutmeg. In a separate bowl, combine the pumpkin puree, sugar, eggs, reserved soaking water, and oil; mix thoroughly with a spoon or whisk. Stir in the pumpkin mixture until it is just moistened. Mix walnuts and raisins in a mixing bowl. Fill a 9x5-inch loaf pan halfway with batter.
4. Bake in the preheated oven for fifty to fifty-five minutes, or until a toothpick inserted in the center comes out clean. Allow it to cool in the pan for fifteen minutes before transferring to a wire rack to cool completely.

PUMPKIN BREAD WITH RAISINS AND PECANS

Preparation: 15 Minutes

Cook: 30 Minutes

Servings: 10

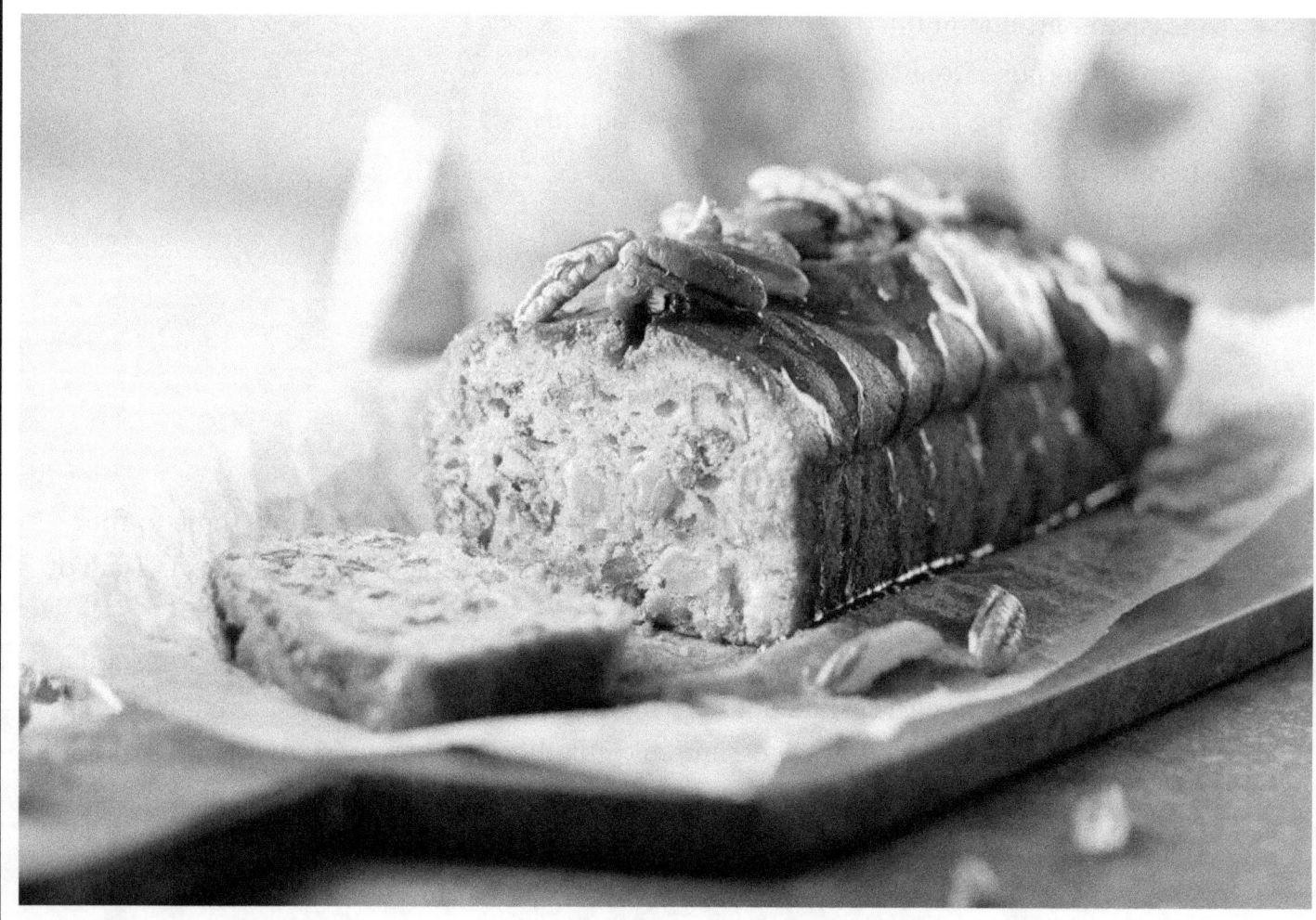

The orange juice gives this moist and tasty pumpkin bread a subtle zing. You can replace the raisins with dried cranberries or blueberries and the pecans with walnuts or other nuts to add variety.

Nutrition

Calories: 262 | Protein: 4.5g | Cholesterol: 61.3mg | Sodium: 592.3mg

Carbohydrates: 42.2g | Fat: 9.1g

Ingredients

- 3 eggs
- ⅓ cup raisins
- ¼ cup butter
- 1 cup white sugar
- ¼ cup orange juice
- 1 cup pumpkin puree
- ⅓ cup chopped pecans
- ½ tablespoon pumpkin pie spice, or more to taste
- ¼ teaspoon baking powder
- ½ teaspoon vanilla extract
- 1 ½ cups all-purpose flour
- 1 tablespoon baking soda
- ½ teaspoon salt

Instructions

1. Preheat the oven to 350°F. Grease and flour 2 loaf pans.
2. In a large mixing bowl, sift together flour, baking soda, pumpkin pie spice, baking powder, and salt. In a separate bowl, toss the raisins and pecans with 1 tablespoon of the flour mixture.
3. In a mixing bowl, cream together the sugar and butter with an electric mixer until creamy. Blend in the pumpkin puree, orange juice, eggs, and vanilla extract until smooth. Blend in the flour mixture slowly and completely. Combine the raisins and pecans in a mixing bowl.
4. Divide the batter evenly between the two loaf pans.
5. Bake for thirty to forty minutes in a preheated oven until hard and tops spring back softly when lightly pressed. Before serving, remove the pan from the oven and cool fully on wire racks.

ORANGE PUMPKIN LOAF

Preparation: 30 Minutes

Cook: 1 Hour

Servings: 12

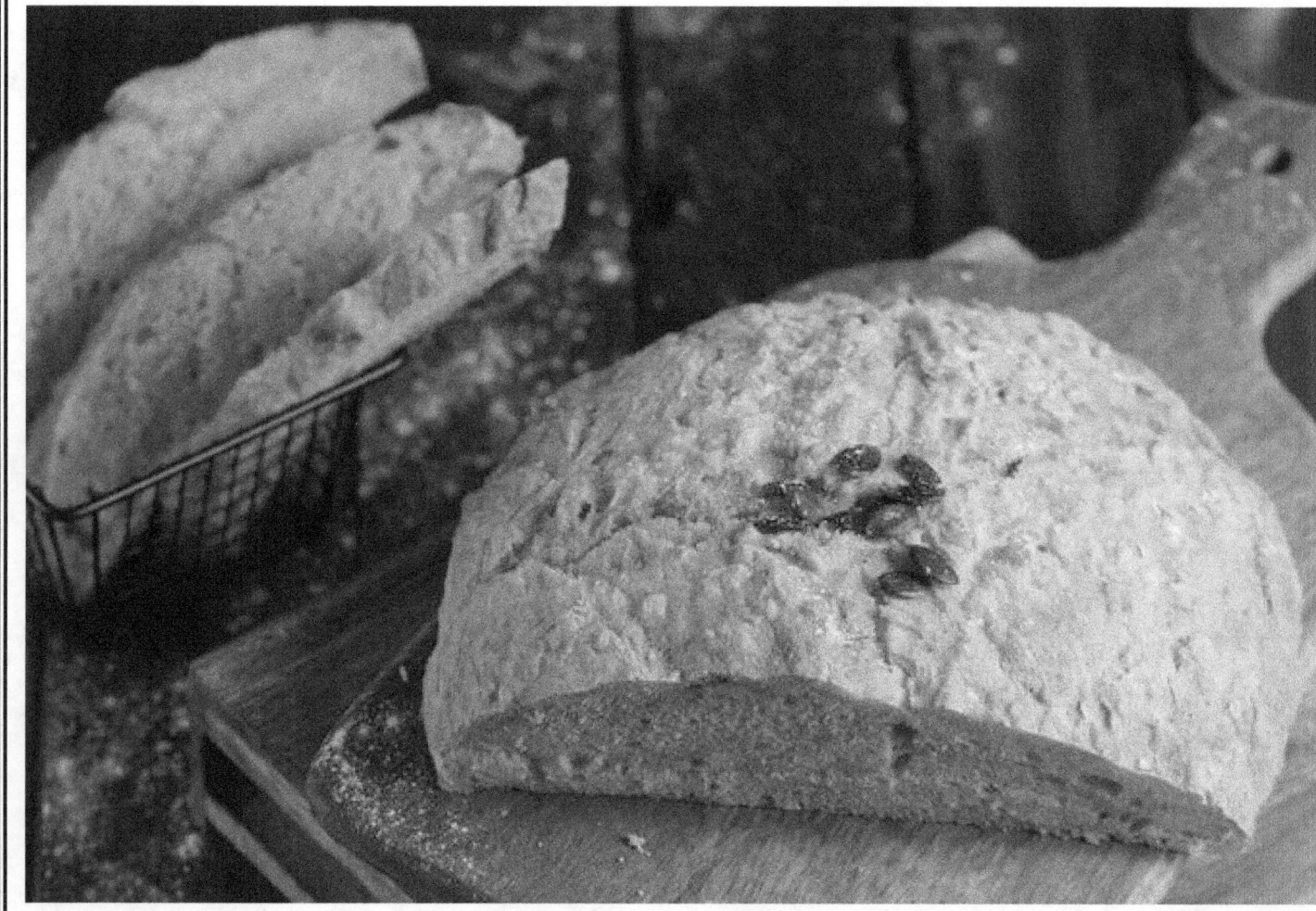

This luscious loaf can be served with an orange cream spread, butter, or plain. Try replacing the raisins with dates for a different flavor.

Nutrition

Calories: 286 | Protein: 4.6g | Fat: 9.5g | Cholesterol: 44.6mg

Sodium: 369.4mg | Carbohydrates: 47.9g

Ingredients

- 2 eggs
- ⅓ cup water
- 2 cups all-purpose flour
- 1 cup canned pumpkin
- 1 ⅓ cups white sugar
- ½ teaspoon baking powder
- 1 teaspoon baking soda
- ½ teaspoon ground cloves
- ½ teaspoon ground cinnamon
- ½ cup chopped walnuts
- 1 large orange
- ½ cup chopped raisins
- ⅓ cup butter softened
- ¾ teaspoon salt

Instructions

1. Preheat the oven to 350 degrees Fahrenheit. Grease a 9x5-inch loaf pan.
2. Remove the seeds from the orange and cut them into wedges. In a food processor, combine the orange, peel, and all, and process until smooth. Set aside after pulsing until finely minced.
3. Cream butter and sugar together in a full of water bowl until creamy. One at a time beat in the eggs, then add the pumpkin, water, and ground orange. Combine flour, baking soda, baking powder, salt, cinnamon, and cloves in a bowl and mix. Stir just until the batter is moistened. Combine the nuts and raisins in a mixing bowl. Pour into the loaf pan that has been prepared.
4. In a preheated oven, bake for one hour or until a toothpick inserted near the middle comes out clean. Allow ten minutes for cooling before removing from pan and cooling on a wire rack.

DOWNEAST MAINE PUMPKIN BREAD

Preparation: 15 Minutes

Cook: 50 Minutes

Servings: 24

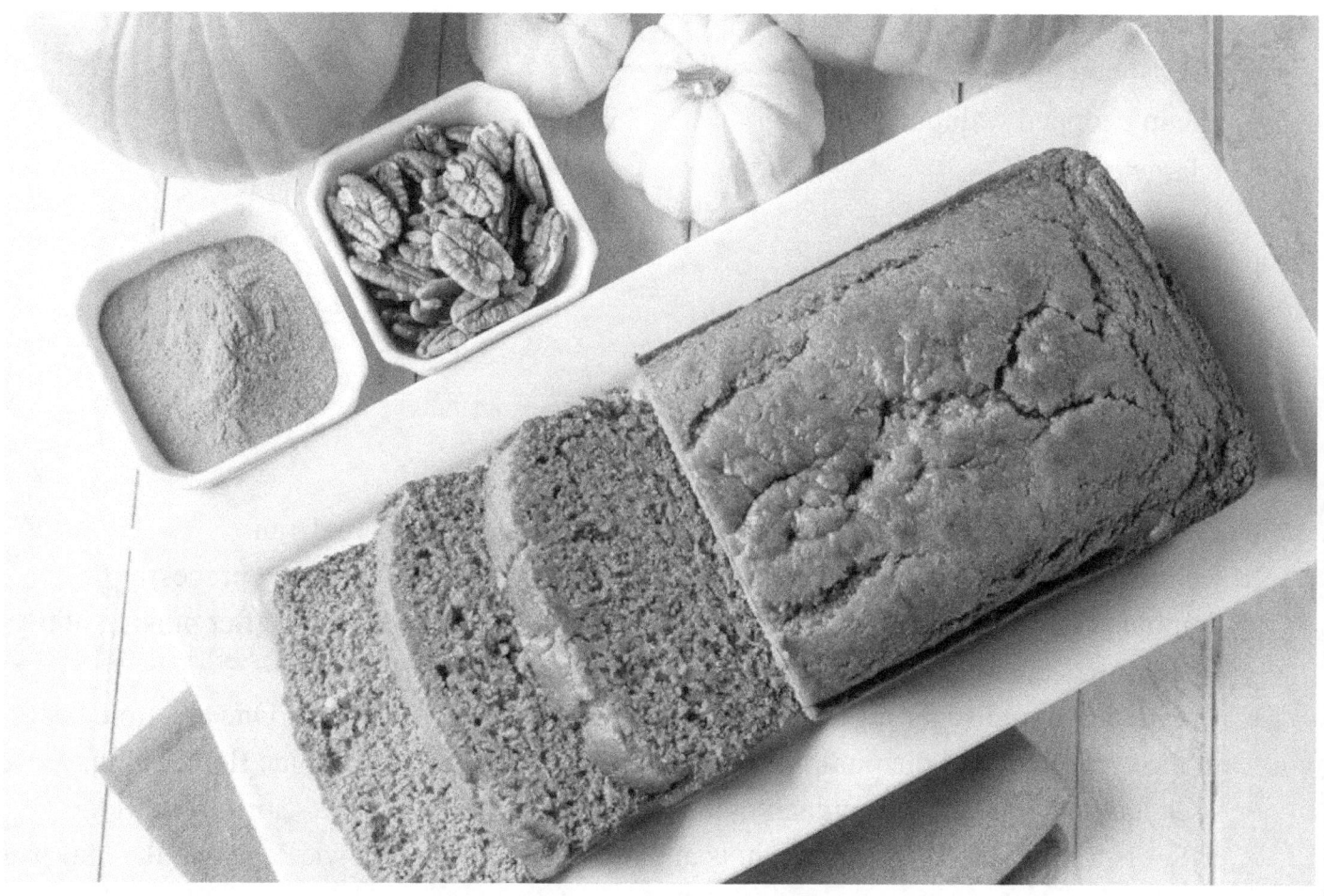

This is a delicious, juicy, and spicy ancient Maine recipe. The bread tastes even better the next day after it has been made. This is a fantastic gift idea for the holidays

Nutrition

Calories: 263 | Protein: 3.1g | Cholesterol: 31mg | Sodium: 305.4mg

Carbohydrates: 40.6g | Fat: 10.3g

Ingredients

- 4 eggs
- 3 ½ cups all-purpose flour
- 1 cup vegetable oil
- 1 can pumpkin puree
- 2 teaspoons baking soda
- 1 teaspoon ground cinnamon
- ½ teaspoon ground cloves
- ¼ teaspoon ground ginger
- ⅔ cup water
- 1 teaspoon ground nutmeg
- 3 cups white sugar
- 1 ½ teaspoons salt

Instructions

1. Preheat the oven to 350 degrees Fahrenheit. Three 7x3 inch loaf pans will be greased and floured.
2. Combine pumpkin puree, eggs, oil, water, and sugar in a large mixing bowl and whisk until well mixed. Whisk together the flour, baking soda, salt, cinnamon, nutmeg, cloves, and ginger in a separate bowl. Mix the dry ingredients into the pumpkin mixture until everything is well blended. Pour into the pans that have been prepared.
3. In a preheated oven, bake for around fifty minutes. When a toothpick inserted in the center comes out clean, the loaves are done.

PUMPKIN CREAM CHEESE MUFFINS

Preparation: 15 Minutes

Cook: 50 Minutes

Servings: 18

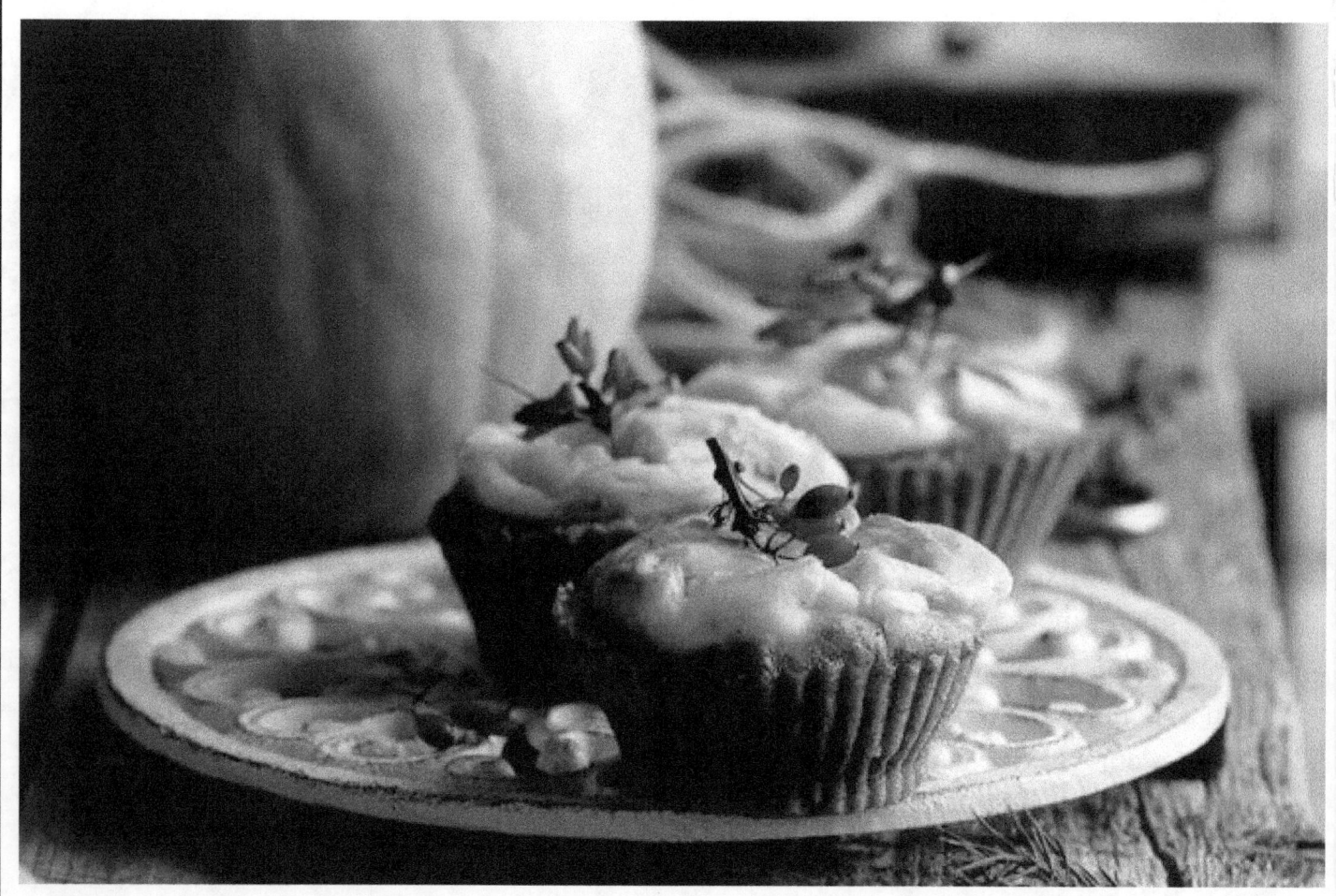

Pumpkin Cream Cheese Muffins are without a doubt one of my all-time favorite muffins! These pumpkin muffins are very delicious and the perfect fall breakfast, packed with spices and stuffed with a cream cheese filling.

Nutrition

Calories: 304 | Protein: 4.3g | Cholesterol: 49.8mg | Sodium: 225.8mg

Carbohydrates: 45.2g | Fat: 12.2g

Ingredients

- 2 eggs
- 2 ½ cups all-purpose flour
- 1 package cream cheese
- 4 ½ tablespoons all-purpose flour
- ⅓ cup olive oil
- 2 teaspoons ground cinnamon
- 2 teaspoons baking powder
- 3 tablespoons brown sugar
- 1 egg
- 3 tablespoons butter
- 2 cups white sugar
- 2 teaspoons vanilla extract
- 1 teaspoon vanilla extract
- 3 tablespoons chopped pecans
- 5 tablespoons white sugar
- ¾ teaspoon ground cinnamon
- 1 ⅓ cups canned pumpkin
- ½ teaspoon salt

Instructions

1. Preheat the oven to 375 degrees Fahrenheit. Use paper liners or grease and flour 18 muffin cups.
2. To create the filling, soften cream cheese in a medium mixing bowl. Combine the egg, vanilla, and brown sugar in a bowl and mix. Set aside after beating until smooth.
3. To make the streusel topping, sift the flour, sugar, cinnamon, and pecans in a medium mixing bowl. Cut in the butter with a fork until it is crumbly. Set aside.
4. Sift together flour, sugar, baking powder, cinnamon, and salt in a large mixing dish for the muffin batter. In the center of the flour mixture, make a well and add the eggs, pumpkin, olive oil, and vanilla extract. Mix everything together until it's smooth.
5. Fill muffin cups halfway with the pumpkin mixture. Then, in the center of the batter, add one spoonful of the cream cheese mixture. Keep the cream cheese away from the paper cup. Finish with a streusel topping.
6. Preheat oven to 375 degrees Fahrenheit and bake for twenty to twenty-five minutes.